EXPERIENCING
PROSTATE CANCER

EXPERIENCING
PROSTATE CANCER

THE FICKLE FINGER OF FATE

Niall Allsop

ISBN 1-49485-722-7

ISBN-13 978-1-494857-22-6

Published by **In Scritto** *Italy in writing*
www.inscritto.com

Cover and book design by Niall Allsop – niallsop@mac.com

Main text set in Sabon
Cover titles and additional notes set in Frutiger

For Dottore Manlio Cappa

... who said I ought to write about it

Acknowledgements

Throughout the experiences that led to the writing of this book two people made it all manageable in ways only they can know. These are:

Kay Bowen and **Dottore Manlio Cappa**

To both I am forever grateful.

In addition I wish to thank the following for their contributions, great and small ...

... in Calabria
Dott. Antonio D'Antonio, Dott.essa Michela Chiarello, Aurelio Gerardi, Silvana Gerardi, Vicki Kelly, Dott. Gregorio Lacava, Denise Milone, Pasquale Piro, Michele Proietto, Dott. Salvatore Ranieri, Dott. Rocco de Rito, Dott. Guiseppe Rizza, Franco Severini, Rosa Stefaniza and Rafaelle Vizza.

At Bios Laboratories, Crotone: Dr Neill Adams, Osvaldo Lucà, Laura Pirillo and Enzo Pugliese.

At Casa di Cura Santa Rita, Cirò Marina: Silvana Aloisio, Patrizia Bortone, Eugenia Trovato and Ermina Ziu.

... in Rome
At Casa di Cura Villa Salaria: Suor'Anna, Dott. Manlio Cappa, Dan Chebac, Dott. Manuel Valentini, Dott.essa Rosella Viceconte ... and all the other nurses and staff.

At the York Hotel: All the staff.

... elsewhere
Dr Christopher Bevan, Deane Logan and Mary Logan.

Contents

Prologue

Sun-dried tomatoes?

People, even people who know about my twisted sense of humor, have asked me about why I chose to embellish the cover of a book about prostate cancer with an image of sun-dried tomatoes.

Well, first of all it's difficult to find an appropriate image for such a subject and you have to admit that there are some depictions of the prostate gland that do actually bear a curious resemblance to sun-dried tomatoes.

On a more serious level, tomatoes (sun-dried or otherwise) are an example of one of the foodstuffs that—according to which website you browse—seemingly have the ability to either prevent, alleviate or contribute to prostate cancer.

The internet is a minefield of conflicting information, a mix of examination, speculation and misrepresentation—most of it meant well, much of it based at best on anecdotal evidence and some of it trying to sell you an idea or a product ... or even both.

Some parts of this book therefore are an antidote to some of that and hopefully will help people find a safe and clear path through the morass of conflicting information out there.

That said, I do not claim that what happened to me is a blueprint for anything; it is no more than an account of *my* experience—both the mistakes I made, the treatment I had and what I can expect in the future.

Also, you cannot fail to have noticed the quirky, tongue-in-cheek subtitle—The Fickle Finger of Fate. This is, I confess, no more than a catchy *double entendre*, a slightly suggestive Rowan-and-Martin-esque catchphrase that stopped short of being too offensive while at the same time alluding to what is usually the first, hands-on, test a doctor performs when it comes to prostate issues.

In reality, in this and every other area, I believe in fate as much as I believe in the tooth fairy.

Finally, although these events all took place in Rome and in the south of Italy they are—apart from the fact that they were also conducted in a foreign language and the initial post-operative 'home' recuperative period was spent in a hotel—a universal story.

Introduction

Surely not another book about having, battling against, coping with, fighting, surviving, beating prostate cancer?

Yes and no.

I did find that I had prostate cancer and I did survive the experience. I don't remember ever 'battling against' it or considering that I was 'beating' it or any other cliché used to describe what was, for my condition, no more than a routine, albeit invasive, course of treatment.

On the other hand I can say that my experience was a little different to most in that, from start to finish, it all happened in a foreign language.

My wife, Kay, and I live in Calabria, the toe of Italy, historically the poorest part of the Italian boot. Despite living here for nigh on four years at the time this story starts, neither Kay nor I were fluent Italian speakers ... and at its conclusion, apart from some newly-acquired medical jargon, we were not much better.

When we moved here in 2008 we expected to absorb the language fairly easily ... we did not allow for the fact that we were both in our sixties and, unlike those forty and more years younger, absorbing a new language was not a natural process for us. Our brains had long since lost their sponge-like capacity, they were no longer the insatiable soakers-up of information they once were. I blame the wine.

Up to a point we do speak and understand Italian, much as a student having studied it for a couple of years might, but not with any depth, not with the nuances that might be appropriate for a medical condition—knowing, for example, the word for 'pain' is not the same as being able to describe it as 'niggling', 'dull', 'sharp', 'sporadic', 'throbbing', 'acute' and so on.

There was also the question of the medical culture in Italy. During those first few years we had, we thought, sussed out how things were done within the state system. But then hitherto we hadn't needed to make much use of it so, when we did, we were in uncharted waters. What came naturally to other Calabrians was, for us, often a perplexing learning curve.

I realize that, even without the problem of language and culture, my experience is both medically unique to me and, at the same time, commonplace; it is no more and no less than what other men of my age have experienced, except that it was *my* experience and in unusual circumstances.

That said, others have goaded me into writing something about it in the hope that it might prove useful to fellow sufferers, if only to make them chuckle now and then. I think my 'goaders' knew I would tell it as it was, the good, the bad and the funny, and that I would avoid the clichés that are the stuff and nonsense of the tabloid approach. They knew too that it is my style to embellish what I write with anecdotes and occasional diversions that, in this case, would be the antidote to what is, after all, a serious subject.

•

By coincidence, I started writing this the very day a much-revered British television personality announced that he had been "battling prostate cancer" for a few months. According to press reports he went on to say that the test for prostate cancer was "if you can pee against a wall from two feet you haven't got it".

If I had used this as my yardstick, I might well have left it too late.

You will have gathered that I do not like the way the media has to embellish the sort of experience I had with the language of war. This tendency has a discernible historic origin when Richard Nixon, the then President of the United States, decided to shift the focus of the press away from other issues, particularly the problematic war in Vietnam, by embracing the concept of a war on cancer and funding it lavishly. The funding part was, of course, an excellent idea.

That was 1971 and by giving cancer a personality it meant that since then very few have ever written on the subject without using words that evoke the idea of battling and fighting, defeating and conquering and, of course, losing.

It is only like that if you choose to embrace that sort of language, if you choose to think of cancer only in such simplistic, combative terms.

Back to that British television personality who seemingly couldn't pee against the wall from two feet away ... of course I have no idea if he actually tried this to test his doctor's theory. Similarly I have no idea if *he* actually said he was *battling* cancer or whether it was just standard tabloid-speak. The point I'm trying to make is that it this sort of language, the language of humanizing cancer, that leads some people to believe that all they have to do is think 'fighting talk' and it will just go away.

Cancer is an illness like many others. Usually you need help to get better; sometimes invasive measures are needed before you get better; and sometimes you never get better.

Awareness and well-trained doctors are the key to getting better ... not belligerent language or alternative hocus-pocus. Which is why, at the beginning of each chapter there is a related quote, generally from a website, on one occasion from a book. The source is also included and, in the case of the websites, all are sites I consider to be generally useful, relevant, thoughtful and unambiguous.

It is because I believe there to be many other internet resources that do *not* fall into the above categories that I have included a chapter on internet-sourced 'information'. Once again this is based on my own experiences and thought processes at the time.

I want to make it clear that I am not a medical professional; I have done many different things with my life but have only ever been involved with medicine as a patient. Nevertheless, I have an enquiring mind and have endeavoured to make the medical information contained in these pages accessible, accurate and unambiguous.

I apologize in advance for any errors I may have made.

At the risk of repeating myself yet again, what follows is not a blueprint for anything. Apart from the next chapter (relating to my medical history), it is no more than an honest, blow-by-blow, account of what it was like for me, a natural-born coward when it comes to such things.

Medical history

Evidence is conflicting about whether previous vasectomy is linked to an increased risk of prostate cancer, but the most comprehensive meta-analysis showed no risk increase.
www.cancerresearchuk.org

When, in August 2008, I told my UK doctor that I was emigrating to Italy the following month, the first thing he did was print out twenty-four pages of notes, my medical history covering the previous fourteen years as a patient at that particular health centre.

Over those fourteen years I had had, as a matter of routine, several digital rectum exams (DRE) to check my prostate gland—in this instance the word 'digital' refers to the use of the finger rather than anything electronic. The only comment I recall my doctor making—other than that everything seemed fine—was that my prostate was smaller-than-usual.

That evening I casually leafed through my medical past, post 1994. For most of that time I had been taking a pill every morning to control my high blood-pressure; occasionally I had had minor ailments, sore throat, odd outbursts of eczema on my palms, a fungal foot infection. In 2003 I had also had one operation, a circumcision and, just a month before in July 2008, an invasive examination, a diagnostic cystoscopy.

I was advised to have the latter because in an earlier routine test small traces of blood were found in my urine ... the doctor who inserted the small camera into my bladder via the urethra announced that everything was perfectly normal is such a way that I felt guilty that I might have wasted his time. In his subsequent letter to my doctor confirming the 'all clear' he also mentioned that my PSA had returned to "within the normal range of 4.0".

This was the first time I had come across the acronym PSA (prostate-specific antigen) ... I knew absolutely nothing about it, what it stood for, what it meant. I leafed back through my notes to check my last blood test earlier that year and there it was again—PSA 4.3.

To my shame, in the throes of preparing to move to Italy, I left it at that, reassured that, whatever this PSA was or did, at least mine was now 'normal'.

I thought back to the two other operations that I'd had pre-1994 and realized that, coincidentally, I seemed over the years to have attracted attention to one particular area of my body, from the waist down and the thighs up.

The first of these was in 1980 when, by choice, I turned up at the aptly-named Love Clinic—named after somebody called Love—to have a vasectomy. It was here that I first evolved the theory that when a doctor tells you that there 'might' be some pain or discomfort or discoloring, he or she generally means that there *will* be some pain, discomfort and/or discoloring.

To be fair there was little pain, only a modicum of discomfort but it took me a little while to get used to the black testicles and to walk without giving the impression that I'd just got off a horse after a long day in the saddle.

•

Two years later, after my then doctor had misdiagnosed shingles, I was back in hospital for emergency surgery to alleviate the excruciating pain of an anorectal (or perianal) abscess; yes, that part of the body again, albeit the back side.

This was the first hospitalized medical treatment I'd ever had through necessity ... though, come to think of it, I did think the vasectomy was necessary at the time.

For those not conversant with the finer details of the anorectal abscess, it is an abscess deep in the buttocks close to the anus and something which has to be treated with the surgeon's knife rather than antibiotics. A deep incision was made to the root of the abscess and the exudate allowed to drain but the incision was not closed as the wound had to heal from the inside out. To assist this the incision was packed with a narrow dressing folded concertina-like. This packing had to be changed every day for about a month or until the wound had healed over.

I was not looking forward to the daily unpacking and repacking and it was while lying in my hospital bed contemplating this prospect that I hit upon something that kept me in good stead then and again more recently ... I 'chose' the nurse that I wanted to unpack and repack.

There are nurses and nurses, just as there are people and people, and homing in on one that the Italians would call *simpatica*—I'm assuming a female, male would be *simpatico*—is, for me, an important part of coping with all that invasion and anticipated pain. I use the Italian word for, though it normally translates as 'nice', it embodies other notions of kindness, caring, accessibility and empathy which, when you're contemplating someone packing a dressing into a hole in your backside, is exactly the sort of person you're looking for.

The following episode will serve to illustrate what this so-called 'packing' involved.

I'd had the surgery and the incision was packed with the concertinaed dressing; a small length of which—the nurse called it the 'wick'—hung from the hole. I was told that the best way to get used to the unpacking and packing process was to remove the first dressing myself and that the best place to do it was in the bath ... I was to take a bath, pull the wick to extract the dressing, and then soak myself again to wash out the wound. Back in the ward, a nurse would then repack with a fresh dressing.

I went for my bath and began to extract the dressing as instructed. I tugged on the wick and the narrow, blood-saturated lint started to exit my backside and, like a magician pulling silk scarves from a hat, it went on, and on ... and on. When finally it came to an end, I was able to drape it along the two top edges of the bath and even then it dangled down a little bit ... I'm guessing it was over two metres long (around seven to eight feet in old money).

Gingerly I sank back down into the water which was slowly turning a deep red; I was mesmerized by my handiwork, marvelling at how all that blood-stained dressing came to be crammed into my backside when my concentration was interrupted by a nurse who'd popped in to see how I was getting on.

She wasn't overly impressed by how I'd decorated the top of the bath with my discarded dressing and, shaking her head, quickly gathered it up in a green paper towel and threw it into the waste-bin. She suggested I empty the bloody water and soak for a short time in fresh water before returning to the ward where I would have my wound repacked.

Later, as I was putting on my dressing gown, I thought I ought to share with Kay what the hospital's medical staff had managed to cram into a hole in my backside so, on the way out, I opened the waste-bin and quickly retrieved the paper towel and slipped it into the pocket of my dressing gown.

Back in the ward I sidled up to my pre-selected *simpatica* nurse—clearly not the one I'd just encountered in the bathroom—and asked her if she would mind sticking several feet of lint into a hole in my backside. She obliged and, as is often the case, the picture in my head of what was happening was worse than any pain or discomfort I may have felt. (Truth be told, over the following few weeks, the only time I felt either of the above was when another nurse performed the deed. My embryonic *simpatica*-nurse radar had done me proud.)

An hour or so later, when Kay came to visit, I checked that nobody was looking and, as I surreptitiously retrieved the paper towel from my dressing-gown pocket, whispered, "You'll never guess what was up my backside ...".

Kay leaned across guardedly as I unwrapped my little green treasure trove to reveal ... a cigarette butt and a broken match.

"You're right", she said, "I'd never have guessed."

●

Everything went fine 'down there' until a few years into the new millennium when I realized that—and I apologize in advance if any of this brings tears to anyone's eyes—when I realized that my life-long inability to pull back my foreskin was increasingly causing me some discomfort. There was also the risk of infection and my doctor referred me to a specialist who advised me to have a circumcision.

I recalled that in my teenage years one's ability, or lack of it, to retract the foreskin seemed to be an impassioned topic of conversation among us boys of a certain age. I was told—and therefore believed it to be so—that if your foreskin couldn't be retracted by the age of eighteen then the man whose unenviable job it was to check on such things would have to force the issue. As I understood it, the tool of his trade, so to speak, was a razor blade.

The friend who told me this tale had just succeeded in pulling down *his* foreskin and in so doing, it seemed, ensured that the razor-blade-yielding foreskin-checker would never darken his door. I listened intently as he explained how, every evening for a couple of weeks, in the privacy of his bedroom, he had forced his foreskin back a little further until that fateful night when, with great relief and considerable discomfort, he managed to do the deed.

I remember vividly his reenactment of the scene: I can still hear the shriek of pain he let out to conclude his tale and picture his worried mother calling upstairs to check that he was alright.

"I'm fine", he called down to her, "... just reading an exciting book".

Try as I might over the next months and years, and always with an exciting book to hand, I never had the satisfaction of that shriek of pain. My foreskin, it seemed, was non-retractable.

In later life, after I realized that the man with the razor blade was not going to darken *my* doorstep after all, the word 'foreskin' was a word I didn't use a lot. The one exception was retelling a story from American writer Kinky Friedman's book, *Greenwich Killing Time* I believe it was, where he described the boots he was wearing as having been made from a brontosaurus's foreskin. Now *that* was an image to relish and enjoy.

But when it came to losing my, more modest, foreskin, I was not overly enthusiastic, however I was assured it was a normal procedure and that it wouldn't be long before everything would be back in perfect working order.

I wasn't so sure.

Pre-surgery I went through the same rigmarole that always befalls me when someone sticks a needle in my arm in search of a vein to extract blood or sedate me. They invariably start with the right arm and even though I insist that they are wasting their time and that I keep all my blood in my left arm, they still have to have a go. And when, as inevitably happens, my right arm is covered in redundant puncture marks, only then do they wander round to the other side and start again. So I was not surprised when I woke up from just having lost my foreskin to discover that both arms were covered in small dressings; those on the left were what I would have expected, those on the right were all the false starts.

I asked about my foreskin and whether it would be possible to take it home. Both attendant nurses looked puzzled until one just had to ask me why on earth I would want to take my foreskin home with me. I had been rehearsing my answer for days ...

"Because I promised my wife I'd make her a lampshade with it."

Both exploded into uncontrollable laughter and I knew then that they'd look after me.

A week later, another unexpected audience weren't sure what to make of it all. I was supposed to be at the wedding of my niece Gillian in Ireland and, because of the circumcision, couldn't attend. The day before the wedding I happened to send her brother, my nephew Neff, an email which included some references to my recent medical adventure.

The emphasise of said email was to draw attention to the fact that, hitherto, I'd never actually seen what lay underneath my foreskin and how, when I did, it reminded me of the helmet of *Star Wars* baddie, Darth Vader. I understand I went on to embellish my discovery by suggesting that this was clearly where the design for Vader's helmet originated. Neff, bless his cotton socks, took the email to be a modern-day substitute for a wedding telegram and read it out to the assembled gathering.

Apparently the silence was deafening.

For the record, everything did get back to normal but it took a lot longer than I expected and I was wearing loose-fitting clothing for longer than I care to remember.

•

And finally, in this catalogue of nether problems there was the aforementioned diagnostic cystoscopy, the camera up the urethra.

Again the notion of having such an intrusion, particularly on a recently revealed and still sensitive Darth Vader helmet, brought back memories of more teenage angst around such matters.

The associated imagery was as bad, if not worse, than that surrounding the mythical man who specialized in sorting out non-retractable foreskins. This one involved a red-hot needle.

What I was told in good faith was that, if ever I had any infections 'down there' the other man, the one who clearly always carried a Bunsen burner with him, would have to eradicate any such contagion—and in so doing teach me a long-overdue lesson—by thrusting a red-hot needle, of indeterminable girth, up my urethra.

Of course eventually, as with the foreskin man, I realized this was just another scarcely plausible teenage scare story.

Nevertheless it left its mark. Years later, when I discovered a document which indicated that my father had been discharged (an unfortunate choice of word) from the army towards the end of World War One for having syphilis, the image of a red-hot needle flashed across my mind's eye. Even though I should have known better, I could not help myself and momentarily did wonder what treatment he underwent and whether or not it involved such an implement.

It is not surprising, therefore, that I was dreading the urethral camera more than any of my other excursions into the urogenital world. On the day itself, what made matters worse was that I was in a waiting room full of men who looked much more ill that I did and who, it seemed to me, felt even more nervous about what was going to happen than I was. I wondered if that was because they'd had the procedure several times already and therefore knew what to expect?

Fortunately, I was the first to be summoned and less than ten minutes later I walked tall—well, taller—back through that same room of worried men and was able to tell them it was fine; I was fine, the procedure was fine too, much better than my anxious mind and my sensitive Darth Vader helmet had anticipated.

On my way out I couldn't resist hesitating momentarily in the doorway and apologizing to them all for the short delay. I explained that it was all my fault ... the doctor had had to fit a much longer lens than was usual. That brought a smile to a few faces ... puzzlement to others.

As already mentioned, the result of the diagnostic cystoscopy was just as I had anticipated: bladder-wise, I was as fit as a fiddle.

•

So, a vasectomy, an anorectal abscess, a circumcision and a diagnostic cystoscopy under my belt, it never occurred to me that there was anything else 'down there' that could possibly give me a problem. Somehow I had missed talk of the PSA test for possible prostate problems and, even when the term was staring me in the face in my medical notes *and* had been referred to in a letter, I was focussing instead on more pressing matters ... like how to relocate the cat, the fish and the chickens before departing for Italy.

It was just two weeks after the camera-up-the-urethra examination (so much easier to say than 'diagnostic cystoscopy') that Kay and I made the decision to move to Italy and a further month before my doctor gave me those twenty-four pages and fourteen years of medical history, shook my hand and wished me and my bits well.

7.13

Men who report prostate symptoms often undergo PSA
testing (along with a Digital Rectum Examination) to help
doctors determine the nature of the problem.
www.cancer.gov

I have written elsewhere (*Scratching the toe of Italy*) about
how Kay and I ended up as patients of The Good Doctor in
the nearby town of Roccabernarda. And how his only other
English-speaking patient, an American woman, coincidentally
also called him The Good Doctor. His real name is Rocco De
Rito so I shall just call him Rocco from now on.

It was not until early 2012 that Kay and I got round to
having routine blood and urine tests. This was not the fault
of the system it was rather our lack of understanding *of* the
system. A doctor could and would send his patients for such
tests as a means of checking up on specific symptoms but, if
you were generally a healthy specimen and wanted a blood
and/or urine test as confirmation thereof, then it was up to
you to ask for it.

When it came to the crunch, there was actually no need to
involve a doctor at all as most largish towns and cities have

laboratories where you can just turn up, have the tests and collect the results a couple of days later. In our case we got the initial list of tests to have from Rocco and then went to nearby Crotone clutching our early-morning urine samples in an armful of blood. A few days later we were back in Rocco's *studio* (surgery) waiting for him to interpret the results for us.

The one he hit on straight away was my PSA (prostate-specific antigen) level of 7.13 and insisted that I come back to Roccabernarda the following Tuesday and see the peripatetic urologist at the local health centre, called an ASL (*Aziende Sanitarie Locali*). Rocco didn't raise any dramatic alarm bells but nevertheless he wanted to have it checked as it was above the magic number 5.0.

It was three and a half years since I had read about my PSA level having returned to "within the normal range of 4.0". In those three and a half years I had had no sense that there was anything wrong. (In Italy 5.0 seems to be the break-off point, in other countries it is 4.0.)

The questions I couldn't ask Rocco because of the language barrier, I sought answers to on the internet. Basically I wanted to know what the PSA test measured and whether or not a PSA level of 7.13 was something I should be concerned about.

The answer to the first part was fairly straightforward. Prostate-specific antigen is, I discovered, a protein produced by cells in the prostate gland and the PSA test measures the amount of this protein in the blood. The level itself refers to nanograms of PSA per milliliter (ng/mL) of blood.

So that's what the number is but what does it actually mean? As ever, the internet threw up a series of confusing contradictions— when it came to finding out what *my* number was telling *me*, the waters were more murky.

There were those who swore by its efficacy—*if a man had a PSA level above 4.0, doctors would often recommend a prostate biopsy to determine whether prostate cancer was present*; those who saw it as no more than a useful indicator—*in general, the higher a man's PSA level, the more likely it is that he has prostate cancer*; and those who thought its usefulness could be overstated—*many men with higher levels do not have prostate cancer ... various factors can cause a man's PSA level to fluctuate.*

In other words my PSA level could be no more than a blip in a sea of normality or it could be a portend of something serious. The PSA test itself could not give me any answers, its usefulness was only going to be as a possible indicator that there *may* be a problem. And because I felt in robust good health, I decided that the number itself probably meant nothing but, nevertheless, I should talk to the urologist as Rocco advised and take it from there.

On reflection I was clearly adhering myself to the school of thought that took my apparent good health as the prime indicator and the reality of the slightly high PSA level as a secondary consideration. I had not forgotten the waste of time that had been the camera-up-the-urethra and I felt, as I had back then, that there was absolutely nothing wrong with me. Back then I had been right and I naturally assumed I'd be right again.

On the Tuesday I turned up at the ASL to see the urologist; all I had with me were the results of my blood and urine tests and the highlighted number, 7.13, on page two.

As he opened up a new folder on me, his first and only English-speaking patient, he asked me how I felt generally and whether I rode a bicycle. When I answered 'no' to the latter he asked me if I sat a lot. I said that I did, that I sat in front of my computer more than a lot, particularly when I was writing, and that probably for most of any normal day I would be seated.

He asked me about the other symptoms associated with prostate problems—frequent night-time visits to the bathroom and, associated with this, not really doing much once I got there. He also wanted to know whether, when I was urinating generally, I'd noticed any difference in the 'flow' and specifically if it was less forceful than usual. The response to all of these questions was "No".

He raised his finger and pointed to the gurney in the corner ... it was time for the digital examination, the fickle finger of fate. He repeated what I already knew, that my prostate gland appeared smaller than normal, and confirmed that he could feel nothing abnormal.

Back at his desk he started to make some notes.

Thus far, language-wise I was doing fine though, like many professionals, he made no allowances whatsoever for the fact that I might not have a clue what he was talking about. I have to say that, unless he had a serious hearing problem, he must have picked up that I was neither fluent nor linguistically confident in this situation and I felt it a bit disconcerting that he wasn't more aware of talking to me in a more measured manner.

He started to write his instructions on a four-page card booklet.

As he wrote, he reiterated that, apart from its size, my prostate gland appeared to be normal nevertheless in the meantime I was not to eat or drink five things until he said otherwise: chocolate (no problem), beer (no problem), coffee (problematic but I would cope), spicy cooked meats (more of a problem) and *peperoncini* (chilli peppers and a big problem). He mentioned the last two in a way which assumed that, as a foreigner, I probably wouldn't eat them anyway and was surprised to find that I ate chillies on almost a daily basis.

Of the five, I rarely ate chocolate, had an occasional beer, drank coffee and ate spicy meats regularly and, as I have said, was addicted to *peperoncini*.

He prescribed some medication, which included a suppository, and initially told me that I was to continue with the medications and the dietary adjustments for three months. He then changed his mind, crossed out the three months part and changed it to fifteen days when I was to have another PSA test.

He went on to tell me that I could buy the medication over the counter at any pharmacy or I could go to my doctor, Rocco, and get a prescription for them. As I felt I should keep Rocco up to date with developments, I decided to go to see him the following morning and collect a prescription.

All this I was of course observing upside down as he sat across the desk from me and wrote; it wasn't till I got home that I could properly read my notes for I had just discovered that, in Italy, it is customary for the patient to be the custodian of his or her notes.

The cover of my little booklet, my *Ambulatorio di Urologia* notes, carried the name of the urologist, my name and age and a reminder that I was to bring these notes with me on any subsequent visit. On page two were all the details of my first visit, starting with my PSA level; pages three and four (the back cover) were left blank in anticipation of further visits.

In reading through those notes I now realize that my interpretation of them was ultimately flawed.

But what was not flawed was my observation that this doctor—and probably most others—clearly had two 'hands' when it came to handwriting. The first part of the notes, which included details of his digital examination, and was therefore for *his* consumption, was written in such an illegible scrawl that I had to get my friend the local pharmacist to unravel it for me; the second part, *my* dietary instructions and *my* medication, was written normally and I understood every word. And there was me thinking that doctors had never learned to write.

The nitty-gritty was as follows. As well as my PSA level, the doctor extracted one other piece of information from my blood and urine text results, namely that there were leukocytes (white blood cells) present in the urine sample, normally an indication of recent or current bacterial infection. The latter was never explained to me, although the fact that one of my medications was an antibiotic should have rung some bells.

This was followed by a description of my near-perfect prostate gland as felt through the wall of the rectum by the fickle finger of fate. The characteristics of my prostate were: "... not large, smooth surface, clean edges, soft texture, tissue not painful, normal contours".

This description was followed by the list of foods I was to eliminate from my diet. I was it seemed allowed one cup of (Italian) coffee a day ... this, it seemed to me, was a sop to the Italian psyche, to the fact that most Italian men would find it difficult to go through a day without a single cup of coffee. I decided that, though I too loved my Italian coffee, it would be easier to do without altogether.

Then there was the medication details, a suppository every evening for a fortnight, an antibiotic after lunch for five days and a drug to treat benign prostatic hyperplasia (BPH), the non-malignant enlargement of the prostate. I was to take the latter for three months and, as is the way of such things, this I could not acquire on prescription, I would have to pay for it.

•

Reading through these notes, I felt good. Everything I'd

learned affirmed that my high PSA level was no more than an indication that the level was higher than doctors liked. The fact that I was ticking so many of the lifestyle boxes (in terms of what I ate), led a generally sedentary life, had none of the other symptoms and felt perfectly healthy was clear evidence that this was a false alarm. The thought that my reasoning might have been flawed never crossed my mind. I was totally convinced that, after a fortnight of drug-taking and dietary restrictions, I would have a blood test, return to see the urologist, slap down details of my new, healthier PSA level and be signed off as just another 'blip'.

As you will have guessed, none of this happened ... but that didn't stop me pretending that it did.

7.40 ... and falling?

PSA has different forms. It can either be *bound* (attached to a protein in the blood) or *free* (not attached to a protein). We know from research that the proportions of free and bound PSA are different in men with prostate cancer, compared to men who have benign prostate disease.
www.cancerresearchuk.org

I recall turning up at the clinic (the Bios Laboratories in Crotone which I will call Bios from now on) for the next blood test full of optimism, absolutely sure that the blood now coursing through my veins was of a lower-PSA variety.

When I returned a couple of days later to collect the results, I was dumbfounded—instead of going down as I had expected it had risen to 7.40.

But it didn't take long for me to realize what had happened— the dietary changes I had made just hadn't kicked in yet. Similarly, the prostate cushion I'd ordered to take the pressure off my poor rectum hadn't yet arrived. Another couple of weeks of abstinence alongside the support of a good cushion would soon get my PSA back within the 'normal' bracket.

And this was the gist of my argument when, once again, I

went back to see the urologist in Roccabernarda. He agreed that perhaps it needed a little more time and told me to continue with his dietary recommendations, insert a few more suppositories of an evening and then have another PSA test in a fortnight.

Once again I left believing that my problem—if indeed I had one—was one of diet and/or lifestyle.

•

Meanwhile, back in the normal world of our daily routines, I had heard that a friend of ours had had some prostate problems and so decided to pick his brains.

It turned out that Franco's problems were quite different and in any case had been cured by a Rome urologist, about whom he spoke in glowing language. He even offered me his number but I declined as I was certain that after my next PSA test I would no longer have need of any further advice, let alone a Rome urologist.

•

Once again I turned up at the clinic with what I hoped was an armful of low-PSA blood and when I got the result I was elated. At last depriving myself of coffee and *peperoncini* had done the trick and my PSA was falling. It was now 6.28.

I celebrated with a cup of coffee in the little bar round the corner from the clinic.

Naturally when I next saw my urologist in Roccabernarda, I was full of confidence for, from my perspective, this was now over, the signs were irrefutable, during this last fortnight my PSA had dropped more than it had risen in the previous fortnight. My body was clearly on the way to becoming a non-PSA zone.

My urologist's reaction was not what I was expecting. He said two words, "OK, biopsy".

Truth be told, my conviction that there was nothing wrong with me or my prostate was so entrenched that I hadn't even come to grips with what might be involved in a biopsy ... I just didn't like the sound of the word.

So the puzzlement he saw on my face I think he mistakenly interpreted as shock and abruptly changed his mind—he had read me well and wrote in my notes that I didn't want a biopsy—and instead said we'd give it another fortnight ... and a different suppository.

The fact that my PSA had dropped was apparently irrelevant, basically it was fluctuating either side of seven which itself was considered to be on the high side.

Deflated but stoically optimistic—based largely on the fact that I was not displaying any of the other symptoms of having a prostate problem—I continued with the dietary regime, the suppositories and the drug to treat benign prostatic hyperplasia.

•

Sometime after this and before the next scheduled test, my friend Franco was asking about how I was and suggested that, if I wanted to talk to someone else about it, I should have a chat with his friend Dott. Guiseppe Rizza. He and Franco were part of a small group of senior citizens who could normally be found sitting outside their favorite bar most mornings putting the world to rights. It was late June and at that time of year this particular bar offered morning shade from the hot Calabrian sun.

I decided we could have a more fruitful conversation if I nipped home and came back with my little folder.

Dott. Rizza was a retired local doctor who probably played a part in bringing most Santa Severinese under forty into the world. In retirement he remained a very popular man and his distinctive shock of white hair, genial demeanor and trademark cigarette were frequently to be seen in the town as he continued to give his ex-patients the benefit of his medical knowledge. Two things I already knew about him were that everyone in Santa Severina still thought of him as the town's best doctor and that, even in retirement, he continued to keep up with advancements in medical thinking and practice. I was, I believe, his first new 'patient' in recent years.

Dott. Rizza read my notes and said that the most important thing he'd seen was that my prostate gland appeared to be perfectly normal and that I clearly wasn't suffering from any of the other associated symptoms.

Here was a man who was speaking my language and inadvertently telling me exactly what I wanted to hear.

He went on to explain that there was another blood test I could have, a new test that provided additional information about the prostate. It was called the PSA (free) and he suggested that when I had my next PSA text I should have the other one too.

I didn't realize it at the time, but I was falling into the trap of only listening to the things I wanted to hear. Dott. Rizza was telling me it straight, he was explaining the science and the pros and cons of what the varies tests meant but at the same time I was hearing: new test—more accurate results—there's nothing wrong with you. And, of course the 'nothing wrong with you' part fitted in with exactly how I actually felt.

It being our fourth summer in Calabria, I was aware that everything wound down during the hot weather so I asked Dott. Rizza to tell me whether, in his experience—and, if after I had the next round of tests in a fortnight, the results remained inconclusive—it would make sense to continue with the dietary restrictions and have another test at the beginning of September and take it from there.

He said it sounded like a reasonable plan but that, if the September test showed that the PSA level was rising, then I should do what my urologist suggested. He went on to say that he did not know this particular urologist and mentioned another name to me, the same man that Franco had talked about a few weeks earlier.

On reflection, the fact that I recalled this conversation suggests that I was probably preparing the groundwork for a 'second opinion' option at some future date.

•

In the past, when a doctor said you needed a particular treatment, then that was that. These days there appear to be options, options that are, in one sense, self-prescribed by browsing the internet. If you don't like the sound of having a biopsy, then there are dozens of websites that will tell you that you don't need one, that a biopsy is not always conclusive, that most turn out to be negative, that they can cause infections. There are dozens more that will tell you there are alternatives, from a few dietary tweaks to drinking fruit juice and tea for forty-two days to make it all go away.

For those in the dark about what exactly a biopsy involves, it is an invasive procedure whereby a number of small needle-core samples of the prostate are removed for analysis. It is normally conducted under a local anesthetic and generally a minimum of a dozen samples are taken. That's the simplistic version; all you have to do now is add all the 'coulds', 'mights', 'oftens' and rarelys' to the equation and then you'll be even more confused than you were to start with.

For me it was quite simple ... someone wanted to take a needle to my prostate gland, grab a few bits, analyze them and then tell me what I already know, that I was as fit as a fiddle ... nor had it escaped my notice that the word analyze had 'anal' in it.

And, no, I didn't like the sound of that, I didn't really want anyone taking samples from my prostate, particularly when I knew it was a waste of time, when I knew there was nothing wrong with me.

But was I frightened of the procedure, was this the real reason for my reticence? Well, at the time, I didn't think so. I simply hadn't taken on board the possibility that there was any problem and why would I even contemplate such a procedure when I didn't need it?

At the risk of repeating myself, everything I thought I'd learned about PSA levels, sitting in front of a computer day in, day out, drinking all that glorious Italian coffee and sprinkling all my food with red-hot chilli peppers—ironically known locally as 'Calabrian viagra'—did nothing more than convince me that I was a hundred percent fit, a fine figure of a man, no less.

•

So, a fortnight on from that first mention of the B-word and still observing the dietary tweaks and inserting my new suppositories each evening, I had another blood test.

Naturally I was expecting the downward trend to continue but instead it rose once more to 7.37. Not quite as high as it had been, but almost, and clearly not inclined to drop as I had hoped ... and expected. Perhaps my urologist was on the right track, after all.

I spoke again with my friend Dott. Rizza, showed him

the results and checked once more with him that it wouldn't be fatal to wait and have another test at the beginning of September and, if nothing had changed, I would consult again with my urologist.

You will have noticed that I have neither named nor said much about the urologist I saw at this time. For whatever reasons I did not take to him; we just didn't gel. Even now I cannot picture him; if I were to pass him on the street, I probably wouldn't recognize him and I normally never forget a face.

Now, whether this was because he didn't seem *simpatico* or he was not saying the things I wanted to hear or because he seemed in a rush to get his biopsy needle out, or a combination of these, I'm not sure.

I think I already knew back then that, were I to need some sort of intervention or treatment, then I would probably seek it elsewhere. By which I don't mean that I didn't think he was competent or that his diagnosis might not be well-founded, only that he wasn't my urologist of choice, he didn't make me feel comfortable.

The internet

Many men with small cancers will not benefit from treatment, because the cancer grows so slowly that it will cause no problems. But it isn't yet possible to determine which prostate cancers will grow rapidly, making treatment decisions very difficult.
www.fhcrc.org

Hearing the B-word had inspired me to step up my research on the internet, even though I already knew that I was unlikely to get anything more substantial than a feel for what would be the right way forward given my particular circumstances.

I have always considered myself fortunate in being able to sift through such information and at the same time separate the wheat from the chaff. I call it my bullshit-button ... everyone using the internet or reading the tabloid press should have one.

Let me give one straightforward example ... it took me no more than twenty minutes to go from that initial twinge on my bullshit-button finger to my ultimate conclusion regarding what I had read on one such website.

A man, supposedly a prospective client of the site, posted the following in support of the arguments of a particular 'natural' health company selling cure-all products for everything from cardiac to prostate issues. He wrote: "I did some research and found that the person that invented the PSA test does not know his own PSA ..."

From this and the rest of his 'observations', it was clear he was trying to discredit the PSA test and, in so doing, make a better case for not having a biopsy. Whether or not what he wrote was true, is irrelevant—the purpose was clear and was the sort of pseudo-argument that is of no help to anyone.

Of course the PSA test of itself cannot tell whether or not you have prostate cancer or any other prostate-related condition ... if it could, then there would scarcely be an outlet for such crass remarks. The test doesn't claim to be any more than an indicator that there *may* be a problem so, ultimately, its result has to be looked at in the context of other known indicators.

And this is the crux of the issue ... what happens when there are no other obvious indicators (as in my case) except that your PSA level continues to rise? What happens when, say, you've had a biopsy that showed nothing untoward and still your PSA marches steadily upwards? It is these sorts of dilemmas that other people feed off for they know how easy it is to engulf an inexact science in confusion ... and, of course, it is then in their interests to thrive on that confusion.

Unfortunately for the man (or woman) trying to find straight answers to straight questions the trail can so easily lead them up many a blind alley and onwards and upwards in ever-decreasing circles or, worse still, into the hands of the charlatans.

So, back to the aforementioned man and his thoughts, rational or otherwise, on Richard J Ablin, the man who discovered the prostate-specific antigen (PSA) ... I don't like loose ends and because I could almost smell the bullshit emanating from this particular website, I did some follow-up research on its claims. The site itself was pretty dynamic and its pseudo-professionalism was gilded with just enough medical credentials, smiling faces and the colour green to seduce even the most seasoned skeptic.

It was a nut much easier to crack than I anticipated; I did a search on the name of the site's 'star' doctor and instantly it popped up on another site called Quackwatch (no prizes for guessing its general ethos) where I found details of a court case brought against said doctor's clinic (not in the field of prostate-related medicine, it has to be said). After the claim was settled out of court (in the plaintiff's favour) the name of the clinic miraculously changed and the same doctor also popped up as the front to another clinic in another part of the country.

Naturally, as is the way of things these days, this particular site had over a thousand 'like' ticks on its FaceBook link, exactly the right sort of number to attract the gullible.

Generally speaking, the English-speaking world is increasingly litigious in nature; if you write, speak or post ill of someone—particularly by calling them a quack or a charlatan or a peddler of bogus wares—and they think it unfair, then there's a good chance you might find a solicitor's letter on your doormat. So, is not the contrary also likely to be true? If no such letter arrives is it not probable that the object of your unkind words does not want their claims, their livelihood, to become the focus of too much scrutiny?

This is something I always bear in mind when I browse the internet ... if I come across a claim, I believe to be, at the very least, dubious, I start to widen my search and never cease to be amazed at what crawls out of the woodwork.

I'm not for one minute saying that the medical fraternity has all the answers ... nor would I expect them to say so. But they are generally accountable and the drug and medications they use have normally been subject to detailed, double-blind testing and scrutiny. The same cannot be said for the sorts of potions that have catchy names and claim to have 'a breakthrough solution'.

Nor do any of these potions alleviate or cure prostate cancer as they sometimes appear to claim. When you read the detail all they actually claim is that they might have some effect on slowing down the onset of benign prostatic hyperplasia—this is enlargement of the prostate gland that can lead to restricted urine flow. They do not cure or alleviate prostate cancer.

•

Now back to all those tomatoes on the cover of this book.

When I first showed my friend Dott. Rizza my list of forbidden foods and drinks he told me that he would have added tomatoes to the list as there was some evidence that they too could affect the PSA result. You will not be surprised to hear that I returned to the internet to check this and found that men should eats lots of them, avoid them altogether and that they made no difference to anything.

So, today, writing this, I took another look ... I searched 'tomatoes and prostate cancer'.

On page one I discovered that "Frequent consumption of tomato products may be associated with a reduced risk of prostate cancer ..."

Further down the same page of search-engine hits, there

was this, "The vast majority of studies show no association ... whether foods that contain lycopene—the nutrient that puts the red in tomatoes—actually protect against prostate cancer.

And on page four I found that, "A Canadian study has found an association between tomato intake and prostate cancer risk".

When my wife and I were preparing for our move to Italy back in 2008, it will not come as a huge surprise that, from time to time, we used the internet as a means of finding out useful information.

It was at this time I realized I had an effective bullshit-button and that much of what I was reading was no more than people moaning and complaining and very little of it was constructive or relevant. It was then that I discovered a quick way of separating the wheat from the chaff ... I checked the date.

Take the three 'tomatoes and prostate cancer' examples above, one is dated 2002, one 2008 and one 2012; unfortunately most internet search engines do not sort by date unless you tell them to do so and in this case the number one hit was the one written over eleven years ago, the one saying that eating tomatoes reduced the risk.

The one that said there was no association between tomatoes and prostate cancer was dated 2012 and was part of a considered article by the high-profile and respected Fred Hutchinson Cancer Research Centre. The one extolling the benefits of tomatoes was, in fact, the oldest while the one dated 2008 was the one giving the opposite point of view.

•

The bullshit-button is not solely confined to websites pushing alternative remedies ... the written word can be equally confusing and these days this too is often accessed through the internet where you can usually read extracts of books before buying.

Take this book, for example, where generally I am relating the story of my prostate cancer, the events as they happened. But here I am pointing a finger at the internet and just about to do the same at some books. I'm doing this because it was a part of the process that I went through; I am not saying I had the only medical intervention available, I'm saying this is how it happened to me.

Unfortunately (some might say 'fortunately') the English-speaking world—and particularly the United States—has, through the internet and books available on the internet, a surfeit of information available to it. The Italian psyche has not yet picked up on some of the more commonplace claims for miracle cures for this, that and the other that have no medical foundation and rely on people's fears and gullibility to peddle their wares.

If television adverts are anything to go by, then sadly this is beginning to change but, even if it does escalate, the fact that so much of this stuff is available only in English will always offer some protection. On the other hand, Google and Bing translations might improve so much that this stuff will soon be knocking at everyone's door.

So, back to the written word. I have a technique for assessing, for example, the reviews of restaurants or hotels on Trip Advisor ... I compare the number of five-star reviews with the one-star ones. Most restaurants will have the odd bad review but if a restaurant has, for example 100 five-star and 35 one-star then that is a highly unusual balance and I, for one, would probably not eat there.

So when I came across a book called *Prostate Health in 90 Days*, I looked at the reviews, and particularly the balance between five-star and one-star, and found it was similar to the balance mentioned above. But I was already uneasy ... the title really annoyed me for it had the sort of ring that preyed on the worried and the gullible.

Nevertheless, being fair-minded, I started to wade my way through the reviews but, after I had read a number of from both sides of the spectrum, my bullshit-button finger was getting twitchy. I was about to hit the delete button but decided to give the author, Larry Clapp—sadly a name open to all sorts of mischievous interpretations—temporary benefit of the doubt and did some more research.

I discovered that Larry had absolutely no medical qualifications whatsoever and that, despite following his own advice, he seemingly died of prostate cancer. I say 'seemingly' for at first the cause of death was shrouded in mystery ... royalties for a book advocating prostate health in ninety days might well dry up if it is suspected that it didn't work for the author. But when I read a moving review of his book by the widow of another man who also followed Larry's advice that was enough for me.

So I'll let 'Nettie', the aforementioned widow, have the last word. The emphasis is hers, not mine:

"Both my husband and his brother tried this diet and followed it perfectly. It did not cure either of their prostate cancers and they both ended up having other treatment ... TOO LATE FOR MY HUSBAND thanks to him believing this crap and wasting the time. Use common sense. Diet may help in preventing prostate cancer but IT DOES NOT CURE CANCER ... Miracle cures like this are a billion $$$$ business because cancer patients desperately want a cure. They should all be shut down including Larry Clapp's book."

•

There is one other internet-based source that is readily available to those seeking further information ... the forum.

Forums spring up whenever and wherever there is a special interest group. They can be incredibly useful if, for example, something is going wrong with your computer or your printer or you want to know how and when to plant tomatoes.

The pitfalls are the same as with other internet sources ... you can be reading something that went live in 2002 and is completely out of date or you can be following advice that does not apply to where you live ... you may want to plant your tomatoes in southern Italy but the advice given is from someone based in France or New Mexico.

As you might expect, health issues have spawned many forums and some of these evolve further and become support groups, even lobby groups that tolerate no dissent from their chosen mantra.

I have already voiced my concerns regarding the efficacy of some of the sites that Kay and I used when we were preparing to move to Italy. I admit I am not a forum person—the lack of any FaceBook or Twitter connections is testament to that— but I did refer to one or two such sites when I wanted to find out something specific, something easy to define.

Kay found such forums more useful than I did, indeed there is one specifically for the partners of people diagnosed with prostate cancer.

When I used them I couldn't help but notice that there were almost as many different answers as there were people and, as ever, I needed to double-check and cross-reference. I also noted on several sites that there are some people who seem to have become almost professional, self-appointed 'advisors', other ex-sufferers who seem to spend most of the day replying to other people's concerns. It may be very altruistic, but I'm not sure who is helping whom nor if, in itself, it is healthy for either party particularly when, as sometimes happens, it degenerates into an argument between two people supposedly trying to help a third.

The difference with medical forums is that generally they *are* peopled by those have gone through similar experiences; they are not trying to sell anything and in most cases are doing no more than relate their experiences. Much as I am doing with this book.

Finally, the news media. I am including this under the general 'internet' heading as many people now receive their news information via their computers, tablets or smart phones. The same general principles apply to the printed word and television, except that with the latter there is generally no way of going back to check that you understood it correctly.

The problem is that, in medical areas, the news media generally settles for a headline that is eye-catching, sensationalist even, and thereafter uses words that let them off the hook. Little words like 'may', 'might', 'can' and 'could' that people miss when they read and then often substitute 'will' when it comes to repeating the story.

I tried something random on a reputable news site (the BBC) ... on their search engine I typed in 'potatoes and cancer'. Up until that moment, I had never seen or heard of anything linking these two words—they were a completely random choice. To my surprise, I got a hit (dated 2002) and the headline read, 'Potato to prevent cervical cancer'.

The headline seemed unequivocal so I clicked on the link to find out more about this breakthrough that had somehow passed me by.

These are the first three sentences; the emphasis is mine:

"The humble potato MAY help scientists to protect women from a common sexually transmitted virus that causes almost all cases of cervical cancer.

US researchers HOPE TO engineer a potato that carries a vaccine against the human papilloma virus (HPV).

IN THEORY, this should provide an easy way to spread immunity at the dinner table."

All I wonder is, how many people just saw the headline and the first few words and came away with the notion that the humble potato either prevented or cured cervical cancer?

And the moral of these stories? Check and double-check everything, particularly the web-page's dates, cross-reference all names and claims and be skeptical if the site is also trying to sell you something ... which is always the case when it comes to books. This one included.

You may even get good at it and develop a bullshit-button of your own.

•

That said, there is no doubt that if you are worried about PSA results and prostate cancer, the internet may well be a useful tool but it can also be very misleading, confusing and contradictory, dangerous even. It's like sitting across the desk from your doctor while he or she diagnoses your condition by telling you there are half a dozen different possibilities and then leaves it like that. He or she isn't going to be more specific or more helpful; your job is to guess which one is right and then guess the cure.

Unfortunately, when you are given so many choices, the temptation is to go with the one you like best, the one that is the most benign and fits in with your general state of health and state of mind.

That is, I believe, what I did. And, as we shall see, when I should have picked up on other signals, seemingly unrelated, I ignored them in favor of my original thesis that I was fighting fit and that there was absolutely nothing wrong with me.

All the information and advice I was gleaning from the urologist in Roccabernarda, my doctor friend up in the square and the internet was telling me the same thing ... my PSA results were a blip, a false reading that was nothing more than an inconvenience.

Putting things off

Although most forms of prostate cancer are slow growing,
the disease does have aggressive forms that can spread and
become life-threatening.
www.fhcrc.org

The warm Calabrian summer started to wane. I was still
observing my dietary tweaks and had already decided that I'd
have my next PSA test at the end of the first week in September.

In the meantime my bright blue prostate cushion had
arrived and I copied the design and made myself two more
for a fraction of the price ... so I had one for the car, one for
watching the television and the original at my desk. I don't
know if they did anything useful but, yet again, in my head
they were ameliorating one of the lifestyle issues that the
urologist first mentioned to me.

Another factor was that I was keen to get all this prostate
bother out of the way before my trip to the United States
in early November to research a book about Calabrian
immigrants.

The night before my planned visit to Bios for the test, I
didn't feel too well. I recognized it as the beginnings of a head

cold so, instead of going to Crotone to have my blood tested, I stayed in bed. That was a Friday and I was confident that, as was usual for me, I'd shake it off over the weekend and be back to normal by early in the following week when I would have my PSA test.

September was going to be a busy month. We were expecting a friend, Steve—an ex-client of mine—from England for a few days and, later in the month, another couple from England, friends of Kay, would drop by and maybe join us at a Calabrian wedding.

Unusually, my expected speedy recovery did not materialize and Steve spent a few bleak days in Santa Severina without his usual drinking partner who had confined himself to bed. I kept thinking I was on the mend but kept relapsing and getting worse between short spells of feeling reasonably fit. Our other guests came and went and luckily caught me when I was enjoying a few days of relative normality.

As September wandered into October, I was focusing on getting better for my trip to the States. I had never felt this poorly for such a long time in my entire life and had now developed a cough that, though not especially painful, sounded much worse than it was. Later our neighbor in the apartment above told me she used to cry when she heard me cough because she thought I wasn't going to survive.

At no stage did I ask myself why this had gone on for such a long time; why my usual resilience to such things had not kicked in. I kept telling people I had never been ill like this for such an extended period—now six weeks—and could scarcely believe it had been so long. It never occurred to me that my body, my immune system, might have been busy trying to cope with something else. I even had to cope with people telling me I should be eating more *peperoncini*, the local remedy to all maladies.

Of course all thoughts of having another blood test simply evaporated—all I wanted to do was be fit enough to get on that plane to New York and to be certain that I could last the distance (a little over three weeks) by myself while I was there. My itinerary was potentially gruelling: twelve flights in total and visits to New York, New Jersey, Illinois, Wisconsin and New Mexico.

When I finally left I knew I was not as fit as I would normally have expected to be but I was also pretty certain I could just about get away with it. And I did.

•

Back on Calabrian soil my priority was making a start on the new book while things were still fresh in my mind and—apart from the brief annual diversion that is the December-January holiday season and a short February trip to visit family and grandchildren in Ireland—this is how I spend the next few months. Most days I did little more than sit on my blue prostate cushion and work at the computer.

That said, for much of this time I had two other health-related issues on my mind.

The first actually started just before I went to America and was a dental problem. For a number of years I had worn partial dentures on both upper and lower jaws which I found both irritating and unsightly. Then, just three days before I flew to America, the gums below my lower front teeth appeared to suddenly drop to reveal a nasty brownish stain just above the 'new' gum line. Try as I might, I couldn't clean it off and as a result I was very aware of it while I was in America, the land of shining white teeth.

When I returned to Calabria I became even more aware of it and rarely opened my mouth in company unless I had to.

Then, for almost a month, either side of Christmas, I also lost much of my hearing; it felt like my ears were full of water and was very debilitating. Despite several visits to The Good Doctor and trying different kinds of eardrops, I discovered it was a sinus problem and soon everything returned to normal.

I mention both these for two reasons. First of all, in retrospect of course, both may—or may not—have been indications of other problems, namely that I was succumbing to things I would normally have brushed off, that my body was more preoccupied with trying to fight off something else. And secondly that both of these health diversions were diversions also in the sense that they took my mind off the other issue ... that I ought to have a PSA test as a matter of urgency.

When I returned from Ireland, for example, I had intended to go for a blood test but instead got side-tracked into trying to sort out my teeth. I had decided the time had come for drastic dental action, and was seeking, via the internet, a dentist in one of the old Eastern Block countries. I knew that the cost of extreme dental work, such as I was contemplating, was considerably less there but also of a very high standard.

I eventually settled on a father-and-son clinic in Rovinj in Croatia and arranged to visit them in mid-March for the first round of treatment. In retrospect it was ironic that here I was, a dental tourist in Croatia dealing with an issue which was, in some part, cosmetic while at the same time hanging over my head there was another more pertinent issue that remained unresolved.

Finally, in early April 2013, nearly seven months later than planned and eleven months on from my first PSA result, I turned up at Bios for that long overdue blood test.

Moving forward

During a digital rectal exam (DRE), the doctor determines
the size and consistency of the prostate, feeling for bumps,
irregularities, soft or hard spots, or other abnormalities. The
doctor also examines the wall and consistency of the lower
colon/rectum

www.cancer.net

I was having a restless night.

I was replaying the scene at Bios when I went to collect my
results. Enzo, the man I usually dealt with on reception, got
up when he saw me come in and returned with Neill Adams,
an English doctor, who worked in the laboratory—but not
normally with the public—and whom I'd bumped into a
couple of times on my several visits the year before.

Enzo handed Neill an envelope, which I knew must contain
my test results, and Neill took out the folded paper and came
over to me. He was emphatic.

"You've got to have a biopsy", he said, "you're PSA is over
ten."

He showed me the result, it was in fact 10.83.

"You need to act quickly", he continued. "Go and see your
doctor."

I knew that these two, Enzo and Neill, had arranged this. As employees of a private company that took blood and urine and analyzed it, their job was an impersonal one. Generally they did no more than give folk a page of numbers; they did not normally consult or advise. But I had got to know both and as they knew that I was neither an Italian speaker nor brought up in the Italian medical culture, they decided to make sure I understood the implications of the results they had just passed on to me. Their concern was over and above the call of duty.

I thanked both and went home to think, to try and equate what I'd just heard with the fact that, despite a winter of ups and down, I once again felt in tip-top shape.

•

Lying in bed that night I realized for the first time that it was possible I had prostate cancer. Despite all my dietary adjustments and my three prostate cushions, my PSA was rising fast and, although I still understood it was no more than an indicator, I resolved to become more proactive and sort it out once and for all.

Note I said 'possible', not 'probable'.

Nevertheless, for the first time I questioned myself and wondered why I had not acted sooner; for the first time I confronted the fact that I might never finish the book I was writing.

For the first time I was frightened.

Still fighting off sleep, I formulated my plan of action. As soon as possible I would seek out Dott. Rizza and show him the latest results. I knew that, whatever he said, he would be a calming influence and put things in perspective. But I also wanted his advice, I wanted to know what he would do and, more to the point, whom he would want to see if he were in the same position.

I think I had already decided that I would not be revisiting the urologist I had first seen in Roccabernarda. This was partly because I didn't feel at ease with him (though I'm sure he was and is a competent urologist) and partly because I felt embarrassed that I had not taken his advice and had a biopsy when he first suggested it. The balance of these two 'partly's has always bothered me for, in all honesty, I cannot be sure which came first ... I sometimes wonder if my embarrassment was the real reason and the 'not feeling at ease' the rationale to explain it away?

Be that as it may, I had decided on a course of action and all I had to do now was find Dott. Rizza. As I have already said, he was actually a retired doctor and, though I knew where he lived, I was unsure of the protocol of just turning up at his door. Better, I reasoned, to bump into him in the square.

A couple of days later our paths did finally cross in the town square and I showed him the results. He asked me about the other prostate symptoms and I confirmed that everything else remained normal. I did not mention the other health issues which I expanded on in the last chapter simply because at the time I did not see any connection between them and the possibility that I might have a prostate issue. And of course there may not have been any connection.

He didn't seem too perturbed by the high PSA level but agreed that I should seek further advice and said that, if it were him, he'd go and see Cappa. He said this in such a way that assumed I should have known who Cappa was. Like if I were a screenwriter with a great script he would have suggested that I should go and see Scorcese or Spielberg.

Dott. Rizza spoke in glowing terms about this 'Cappa' and that he was *numero uno*, the top man in Rome, in Italy, further afield even. And this Cappa also happened to be Calabrian and, every four weeks, he drove down from Rome to Crotone to hold a surgery, to give something back to the community that had raised and educated him. He was trying to find his address book to check if he had a number for Cappa just as our mutual friend, Franco Severini, joined us.

This was one of the things I liked about Calabria, the fact that people generally were open about their ailments and didn't shroud them in whispers and secrecy. When Franco sat down and ordered his coffee, the conversation returned to *my* prostate and Dott. Cappa who, it turned out, was the man whom Franco had seen regarding *his* prostate problem the year before.

Once again, I detected a reverence in Franco's voice when he spoke of Cappa and within seconds he had scribbled his number on a scrap of paper and told me I should give him a call.

Unfortunately—and unknown to me at the time—Franco made a mistake on the number's last digit so I made several fruitless calls before I realized there had to be something wrong; it was therefore over a week before I was able to reach Dott. Manlio Cappa and then I found I had just missed one of his four-weekly surgeries.

That spring Kay and I had two trips to England planned—for the wedding of Kay's daughter in May and of my nephew in June—and, between the two, another trip to Croatia for the second round of my dental treatment. Before I finally got to make that appointment with Dott. Cappa, Kay and I had resolved that, whenever he said he could see me, I would be there—even if it meant missing one or more of our planned trips.

As it happened he was in Crotone on May 11, a week after Amber's wedding and ten days before we traveled to Croatia.

Kay and I drove to Crotone in buoyant mood. I still felt well, so well in fact that we decided I'd go and see Dott. Cappa alone while Kay indulged in a bit of retail therapy. We arranged to meet in a café around the corner from the surgery.

Dott. Cappa's surgery is on the first floor of an old three-story building close to Crotone's market and a few minutes walk from the sea. It consists of a waiting room and a restroom, a consulting room with adjacent examination area.

It is manned by Michele, Dott. Cappa's male nurse-cum-receptionist who was my first point of contact before being shown in to see Dott. Cappa himself.

The genial, softly-spoken, bearded man behind the desk shook my hand warmly and asked what the problem was. I handed him my collection of PSA results and my notes from the urologist in Roccabernarda.

He read it all in silence and asked me about my night-time urinary habits and how I felt generally. I told him that I sat a lot—but didn't ride a bicycle—but otherwise felt generally fit and well. I never mentioned any of my recent ailments as, at the time, I still had no reason to think they might be relevant. I did however tell him about my recent dental trip to Croatia in which he was very interested ... not in connection with any urology issue I might have, but rather as a potential patient himself.

I then had the routine digital examination, another fickle finger, after which he too opened a file on me as he shared his thoughts with me.

He said he had felt something the size of a small pea on the right lobe of my prostate and that I was to come to Rome the following Saturday where he would perform a biopsy at the

Casa di Cura Villa Salaria, a private clinic where he worked. He told me how much it would cost but did not ask whether or not I had private insurance.

He went on to explain that he no longer performed biopsies locally as the analysis of the samples was still done in Rome and it was his experience that they did not always fly well and therefore any analysis could be flawed.

He gave me a list of three medicines I was to start taking in the days leading up to the biopsy—something to reduce the risk of hemorrhage, an antibiotic and Vitamin C; I would continue to take the last two for a short after the biopsy.

He also gave me details of how to find the clinic and told me he'd see me there at ten-thirty on Saturday morning. He said I could now ignore all the dietary stuff I'd been adhering to for almost a year. And finally he told me that, whatever might be wrong with me, it was fixable so I was not to worry ... it would all be fine.

I believed him implicitly.

We chatted a bit about how it was Kay and I had ended up in Santa Severina before he asked me if I'd any questions for him. The only one I could think of was whether or not, on the Monday after the biopsy, I would be fit enough to fly to Croatia for my next round of dental treatment.

"Definitely." he said.

•

Ten minutes later I was sitting in a small café relating these events to Kay. I started with the conclusion ...

"We're going to Rome next weekend."

I explained why and so we immediately started to plan the logistics of it all as we had already booked flights on the post-biopsy Monday from Lamezia Terme (our not-so-local, local airport) to Venice where we would pick up a rental to drive to Croatia.

We decided to drive to Lamezia on the Friday and leave the car there, travel to Rome by train (five hours) and stay overnight in a bed & breakfast a fifteen-minute walk away from the clinic.

We'd stay in Rome for two nights in total and on the Sunday return to Lamezia by train and stay overnight in a local hotel before flying to Venice the following (Monday) morning.

It all seemed doable.

That evening we ate out ... I had my usual tuna-and-onion pizza and, at long last, the icing on the cake, a liberal sprinkling of dried *peperoncini*.

•

Over the next week I had plenty of time to think about what had transpired on my brief visit to Crotone that Saturday.

Not for one second did I ever think that this was going to be any more than a false alarm, that the biopsy would confirm that my prostate was in fine fettle. The fright that I'd experienced when I had the last PSA result had evaporated.

At the same time, not for one second did I think that the biopsy was unnecessary. On the contrary, I really felt I should have it to settle this once and for all so that life could get back to normal rather than having the spectre of these infernal PSA numbers hanging over me.

Above all, I felt I was in good hands. I liked Dott. Cappa a lot; he was, it seemed to me, just an ordinary person who liked to wear a white coat. The fact that every month he made the journey from Rome to Crotone (a round trip of about eight hundred miles on not the best of roads) was testimony to how he viewed his role as a doctor.

He made sure I understood everything and even spoke in English from time to time to consolidate this. He also had an interest in things non-urological. He inspired confidence and I knew that, had he told me to hop everywhere for the next week, I would probably have given it my best shot.

I understood too how it was that people spoke about him with such affection. There was some reverence there too but, above all else, it was affection that I sensed.

Also that week, I sought out Dott. Rizza and Franco to share with them my experience in Crotone. The former confirmed that he guessed that was what would happen and both independently made the same observation.

"You're in the best possible hands." They said as they kissed and hugged me.

I already knew this to be true.

The biopsy

A prostate biopsy is a procedure in which prostate gland tissue samples are removed with a special biopsy needle ... to determine if cancer or other abnormal cells are present. The diagnosis of cancer is confirmed only by a biopsy
www.hopkinsmedicine.org

As planned, we arrived in Rome on the day before the biopsy and on the Saturday morning walked to the clinic.

The plan was that, post-biopsy, we would return to the bed & breakfast by bus—there was a stop just outside the clinic— have a light lunch and just rest all afternoon. I only mention this because that's not what happened.

Being of northern-European stock, we arrived early and waited for about half an hour in the large, bright and clean reception area with its adjacent tidy little cafè-bar. So I had time to contemplate my fate.

I have a strategy for coping with events about which I am apprehensive or when they take an unexpected (negative) turn. I simply think about the time after it's all over.

Take, for example, the time we were lost in Seattle and I (as the driver) couldn't seem to find my way out of the maze of streets and on to the adjacent freeway that would take us back to the bed & breakfast. Instead of panicking, I thought of being in bed and waking up to that wonderful all-American breakfast like the one I'd had that morning. I was certain that's how it would be: that the next morning I would enjoy a similar breakfast, and that somehow this bad moment would develop into that good moment. I just had to find a way to make it happen.

And, of course, I did.

So, sitting there in Villa Salaria, I was naturally a little apprehensive but I knew also that each moment that passed would bring me closer to a pleasant lunch, a rest and a Chinese meal in the evening. Whatever happened in between was a necessary evil and it would pass.

•

The receptionist took me round to Dott. Cappa's small consulting room-cum-office complete with partially screened-off gurney. Dott. Cappa welcomed me and introduced me to his colleague, Dott. Manuel Valentini. I handed him my file having first extracted from it the brochure about the dental clinic in Croatia that I'd promised him. Momentarily both Dott. Cappa and Dott. Valentini, ignored my notes, flicked through the brochure instead, and talked to each other about the advantages of dental treatment in Croatia ... particularly the cost.

Dott. Cappa put his hand on my shoulder and with a sympathetic smile and reassuring words pointed me in the direction of the gurney where I was invited to remove my lower garments.

On a shelf by the gurney I had already clocked a huge hypodermic needle, the sort that I would have expected a vet to wield in the presence of a horse or a cow. I remember thinking that it couldn't possibly be for the likes of little old me. But, of course, it was and its enormous girth was a means of making sure I had enough local anaesthetic for them to proceed with the biopsy.

As I pulled up my legs and held my bits well out of the needle's way, Dott. Cappa got to work with injecting the anaesthetic which he did very slowly, pausing regularly to make sure I had no discomfort or pain. When he'd finished he left the room for five minutes and so I had a chat with his colleague who, like most Italians, was intrigued as to how it was that Kay and I had ended up in Italy, and Calabria in particular. Dott. Cappa returned just as I'd got to the part about the red wine.

Dott. Cappa checked that I was feeling alright and then began. He kept me up to date with the progress of the sample-snatching needle as it approached the prostate and said he would be taking samples from one lobe and then the other. He added that would probably take more from the right—the lobe where he'd felt the pea-like nodule. He confirmed that I shouldn't feel a thing.

He was right ... but he omitted to tell me about the sound. As each sample was taken it sounded a bit like a staple-gun firing, not at all what I was expecting and at the time a little disconcerting. He was right, I felt nothing ... just noise pollution and the picture in my mind of what was happening down there. After each sample was taken, he passed it to his colleague who put in a small phial and off he went again, snatching away at bits of my prostate.

I started to count ... one ... two ... three ... four ...

Then I noticed that he was watching a screen, the back of which faced me. I asked if he was looking at my prostate and he said he was and asked if I'd like to watch too. I nodded and so he repositioned the monitor so that we could both see it ... he was guiding the needle and I was watching its progress and trying to marry up what I was seeing with the sound I was hearing.

It seemed to me that the action on the monitor was just like the scan we are all used to seeing of the unborn child in the womb. I thought I'd lighten the proceedings by asking if he could tell whether it was a boy or a girl. Somehow my attempt at a joke got lost in translation ... they probably thought I was hallucinating.

It was at this point that I lost count of the number of samples he'd taken but felt sure he must have got close to the dozen that I was expecting. I then realized, I never actually asked him how many samples he wanted. And when I did, he told me he'd take eighteen pieces ... he went on say that, as my prostate gland was quite small, taking eighteen samples was more difficult than usual.

He must have been getting bored for the conversation once again focused on dentistry. He asked me if what he was doing to me now was worse, or better, than the dental treatment I'd had in Croatia. (He knew that, for example, in four non-stop hours I'd had seven implants, two sinus lifts, a bone graft and between forty and fifty stitches.) I genuinely had to think about it and found it difficult to equate the two experiences, particularly as one was actually happening to me at that very moment. Nevertheless I said the dental work was worse for I knew it would make him feel better about what he was doing to my poor prostate.

•

The biopsy over, any excess blood—for there was a little bleeding—was wiped away and both doctors gave me a hand to get back on my feet and checked that I could walk reasonably normally. Other than a little stiffness from having been stuck in the same position for nearly half an hour, I felt fine.

Before I finished dressing, I was given a pad to put between my legs to soak up any additional bleeding and told to return to the waiting area, have a coffee and he'd see me again in an hour or so to check that I was fit enough to head 'home'.

As I was about to leave, Dott. Cappa asked me if my wife was with me and, when I said she was, he said he would like to meet her and assure her that it had all gone well.

This simple act of kindness was something Kay and I very much appreciated. He didn't have to do this, it was just something that he instinctively knew would be an important gesture, an indication that he was a human being first, a doctor second. The treatment I had just had was *to* me but *for* us.

Back in the reception area, the introductions over, Kay and I retreated into the little café-bar for a coffee. We found it also had some tables in an adjacent garden and went out to sit in the warm June sun.

I felt demob-happy. I was relieved that it was all over and genuinely surprised that it had seemed less invasive than I had imagined. Back in the reception area I alternated sitting, standing up and walking but the only discomfort I felt was the presence of that extra padding between my legs.

It was approaching lunchtime when Dott. Cappa poked his head into the waiting area and signaled for me to return to his consulting room. There he removed the pad and checked that all seemed well and said I was good to go. I did the hard and dangerous (paid up) and he wrote me out a receipt. As I stood up to leave I noticed a graphic anatomical representation of the male body on the wall behind me and asked him to show exactly what he'd done.

This was, he said, an interesting question because there were several ways of reaching the prostate and he didn't now use the procedure, still the most common in the UK and America, called the transrectal biopsy where the needle goes through the wall of the rectum. As he was speaking he was showing me this on the graphic.

He then showed me how he accessed the prostate gland by inserting the needle through a cut in the perineum, the area of skin between the anus and the scrotum. The biopsy needle passes through the cut and into the prostate to obtain the tissue samples. He went on to say that in most cases this approach gives access to more of the prostate than other methods which meant that there was generally less likelihood of negative results when in fact there was something there.

He maintained it was a simpler procedure and that there was less risk of post-biopsy infection; in addition, after the procedure, patients generally felt better sooner. I felt I was living proof of that for I did feel fine.

I made an appointment to see him again in Crotone in three weeks time—by which time he would have the biopsy results and I would be less dentally challenged—shook his hand, thanked him and rejoined Kay in the reception area.

•

Kay thought we should return to the café-bar to have some lunch but I was keen to get back 'home' and suggested we pick something up on the way. So we left the clinic and walked to the nearby bus-stop to wait

Almost a quarter of an hour into the waiting I realized I'd left the receipt for my treatment on the desk in Dott. Cappa's office so Kay volunteered to return to the clinic to fetch it. While she was away the inevitable happened, the bus came and went. It's called Sod's Law.

Almost a quarter of an hour into the second period of waiting, I was leaning against the pole of the bus-stop, my arm wrapped round it, when I slowly started to descend ground-wards—Kay said afterwards that it was as if I was rehearsing a new slow-motion pole-dancing routine.

Kay ran behind me to try and support me before I became a crumpled heap but, fortunately, a man passing by caught me and supported my weight while I gradually regained my focus on the world around me. Slowly he started raising me upright, pausing several times to check that I was ready to proceed a little further towards the adult world.

At this point another, younger, man appeared who just happened to be a physiotherapist from Villa Salaria and who, when he heard I'd just had a biopsy there, suggested I return to be checked over. At this point a car drew up, a Jaguar no less, and the driver and his wife offered to drive us back to the clinic even though it was no more than a hundred yards away.

So, forty minutes after leaving Villa Salaria, I was back there. Dott. Cappa had left for the day and I was now up on the second floor having my blood pressure taken. It was, as I already had surmised, very low.

The problem was simple, it was five hours since I'd eaten and in the meantime I'd had an invasive medical procedure and, instead of eating at the clinic and/or getting a taxi back to our bed & breakfast, I'd opted to wait for a bus ... twice. My blood-sugar had dropped like a stone and out by the bus-stop I had followed suit.

Basically I should have known better, I should have listened to Kay when she said we should eat something in the café-bar before leaving.

The duty-doctor suggested I go downstairs and rectify that situation immediately and then he'd check my blood pressure again in an hour or so.

It was nearly four o'clock in the afternoon when the taxi dropped us off 'home'. I went straight to bed for a nap, not because of any after-effects from the biopsy as such ... I was just very, very tired.

Post-nap, I decided to check something out on the internet that I'd remembered reading in an extract from a book, a description of the prostate biopsy written by an urologist. After a few false starts I tracked it down in a book called *The Decision: Your prostate biopsy shows cancer. Now what?* It read as follows:

"You've just experienced the anxiety, humiliation and pain of having your prostate biopsied. Since the biopsy you have endured the sight of blood in your urine and bowel movements, blood in your semen, and burning when you void."

Having just had my prostate 'biopsied' I could truthfully confirm that I felt some anxiety (who wouldn't?), absolutely no humiliation and no pain that merited a stronger word than 'discomfort'. At the time I couldn't be sure about the remainder of this emotive list. In retrospect, I recall a miniscule amount of blood in my urine for no more than a day.

In other words, what I'm saying is that I think such remarks are crass and unhelpful to people who are considering having such a procedure ... particularly as they are clearly describing only one biopsy technique. They are also disrespectful to the many doctors who try so hard to limit all anxiety, humiliation and pain.

●

With the upcoming dental trip to Croatia, we would have successfully negotiated two of our three summer excursions. Our next visit to Crotone would settle the fate of the third, nephew and best friend Graham's wedding on June 15 in London.

The results

The pathologist adds together the grade of the most abnormal looking cells to the grade of the most common pattern of cells. They add these scores together to make the Gleason score.

www.cancerresearchuk.org

The trip to Croatia came and went as planned. My smile was looking better and I would return for the final treatment and a full smile at the end of September.

While we were in Croatia I talked to my dentist, Ivan, about my recent biopsy and he told me that his father Željko had had one recently too and that everything was all clear. He went on to say that Željko was advised by his urologist not to drink carbonated water or similar drinks.

This was a new one on me and set me thinking that perhaps every culture has something they associate with prostate problems ... preferably something that everyone really likes.

Almost instinctively, I stopped drinking fizzy water while we were there and even back in Calabria. The power of the unsubstantiated anecdote knows no bounds.

On the following Saturday we headed back to Crotone for

the results of the biopsy. Once again I was in buoyant mood and was not expecting anything more than a firm handshake from Dott. Cappa which would confirm that the biopsy was 'clear' and all was well with my nether regions. My worst envisaged scenario was that I might need some therapy for some related condition.

But it wasn't like that. The social formalities over with, we got down to business.

Sitting across from us, Dott. Cappa shuffled his papers, selected one and placed it in front of Kay and me. It was, of course, in Italian.

"As you will see," he said, "the biopsy showed that you have prostate cancer. On the Gleason Score, 3-4, a total of 7. A moderately aggressive cancer."

He went on to explain how the Gleason Score worked and what the two numbers meant and what the prognosis of their total was. Much of this was shrouded in technical language but both Kay and I knew a little about the significance of a Gleason Score. As this was the recognized system for assessing prostate cancers, I knew we could check out the finer details later—in this instance there were unlikely to be dozens of different internet explanations.

"But the good news is we can make it go away." he continued, "This is what we must do ..."

There followed an intensive session of questions and answers, mostly in Italian, occasionally for clarification, in English. On both sides it was a considered, rational and focused discourse. Dott. Cappa was, it seemed to me, aware that this was something that we had not expected and he was walking us through it with the right balance of information and compassion.

He started by explaining the options and it was clear that he was discounting the first two—radiotherapy and continuous monitoring.

He considered that in my case, given my Gleason score and the increase in PSA levels, a long course of radiotherapy would just be putting off the inevitable and that surgery, post-radiotherapy often came with a higher risk of side effects, particularly incontinence.

He mentioned too that in some Scandavian countries in particular there was a tendency to go through a period of continuous monitoring of the prostate before treatment but that in his experience this could cause additional and sometimes prolonged anxiety. My cancer was, he was sure, only going to get worse and there was no point in pretending otherwise.

He told us that, in his opinion, I needed an operation to remove the prostate gland and that this could be done as a laparoscopic radical prostatectomy by him in Rome.

The term 'laparoscopic surgery' is synonymous with keyhole surgery and it was a term we were acquainted with since a close friend's gall bladder had been removed in this way several years previously. Dott. Cappa explained how it is a less invasive procedure with small incisions in the abdomen through which he can insert the laparoscope (a small tube that includes a light source and a camera) and other small tools. He also explained that there would also be one slightly larger incision (about an inch and a half) through which the prostate would eventually be removed.

At the time, when he was sitting there explaining what he was planning to do to my body, I had no real sense that this was something that was going to happen to me. I trusted him implicitly and never doubted for a minute that the procedure was a necessary evil but in another sense I had detached myself from the proceedings, was observing rather than participating. I was grateful that Kay was there as a second pair of ears.

Having outlined the procedure itself, he went on to explain the most important implications.

I would be without my prostate, the gland responsible for the secretion of most of what constitutes semen. He would also remove the vas deferens and the seminal vesicles both of which would be redundant without the prostate gland.

Depending on what nerve bundles he could save, I would continue to have erections and could climax normally but without any ejaculate—I was already calculating the savings on paper hankies. To aid this whole process I would take a drug called Cialis (a form of Viagra) for up to three months post-operation.

Dott. Cappa seemed confident that the cancer had not spread to the nerves but could not guarantee it. If the worst came to the worst and he had to remove these handy little nerves, then we would be looking at some sort of mechanical aid to retain the erectile function.

After the operation I would have a catheter for up to ten days—during which time I was not to drive—and, after this was removed, would need to wear diapers for as long as took to become continent again. As he would remove some of the nerves that play a part in controlling continence, I would need to relearn how to control urination. I would be returning to my infancy, albeit with a keener sense of the social graces when it comes to urinating in public places even with a diaper.

This, he stressed, varied considerably between patients and indeed was something that the patient could often alleviate by doing appropriate exercises.

Dott. Cappa turned next to the where and the when as these two were irrevocably linked. The procedure could be done at Villa Salaria, a private clinic, or at the Fabia Mater Hospital, part of the *Servizio Sanitario Nazionale*, Italy's national health service. One you paid for (or had medical insurance to cover the cost), one you didn't.

Aware that we had already had experience of the former, he only brought with him information on Fabio Mater, including details of nearby accommodation. He emphasized that, whichever we chose, he would perform the operation using identical equipment. The major differences between the two were cost, the fact that Kay could stay in the same room with me only at Villa Salaria and the timing.

At Villa Salaria, I could have the operation in a fortnight; at Fabia Mater it would be the end of July (about seven weeks) unless there was a cancellation which, he said, was not uncommon.

We told him we were fully paid-up members of the *Servizio Sanitario Nazionale* but that we did not have medical insurance and that we would therefore like to know the financial implications should we opt for Villa Salaria. His subsequent calculation was based on the supposition that we would stay at the clinic for no more than four nights.

We told him we would text and email him our decision regarding the where (and, by default, the when) that afternoon.

Dott. Cappa then produced a list of medications I was to take in the days leading up to the operation. This was similar to the one he'd given me before the biopsy but with one important addition—on the evening before the surgery I had to take two doses of a powerful laxative, two hours apart, and drink two liters (about four pints) of water after each dose. I couldn't wait!

Another list he gave us detailed a series of tests I was to have done before I came to Rome—I was to bring the results of these with me on the day before the operation. These were:

A lengthy list of blood and urine tests
A full body scan (CAT scan) with contrast
A bone density scan
X-rays of the thorax
An electrocardiogram

All of which, at the time, seemed relatively straightforward. Our main preoccupation in the next hour or so was going to be the cost should we go for the Villa Salaria option.

All three of us knew we'd covered a lot of ground in a relatively short time and Dott. Cappa stressed that we could always contact him if we wanted any additional clarification or had any concerns.

He reiterated that, in my case, this treatment was the only viable option and that it was a procedure he had been doing for many years and he was confident that the prognosis was excellent. He added that, if we opted for Villa Salaria on June 22, then we would become part of an international day of laparoscopic radical prostatectomys as he was doing another such procedure that same day on a Romanian man. I could see he quite liked that idea.

It was time to leave but just before we did Dott. Cappa said he knew I had cancer the first day we met but that he had to have confirmation from the biopsy results. It was almost as if he was apologizing for having had to put me through it.

It was two slightly shocked people who headed back to Santa Severina. Nevertheless, en route we discussed the options and the implications and made our decision.

Of course one of the things we looked at—albeit briefly— was the possibility that Dott. Cappa was advocating surgery as this was his how he made his living. But we soon discounted this as all the things we already knew about him and his reputation, and our personal experience of him, told us that this was not the case.

Once home, I emailed and texted Dott. Cappa with the same information ... we wanted to be part of the international laparoscopic radical prostatectomy festival at Villa Salaria on June 22. We would arrive in Rome on the afternoon of Thursday June 20.

The most important decision out of the way, we had a hug and a cry before focusing on the many things we knew we had to do over these next few days. We were heading into uncharted territory but we knew we'd get through it ... after all, we'd been here once before many years previously. Only this time the tables were turned.

•

Before I started checking on trains and searching for a hotel, my initial priority was to email a friend in England who also had had prostate cancer (with a PSA of over 90) to tell him my news ... and invite comment.

Next I set about checking out the implications of my Gleason Score of 3-4. I knew that Dott. Cappa had been stressing the difference between 3-4 and 4-3 but the subtleties of the distinction in Italian had passed me by.

The numbers refer to the most common tumor pattern found in the samples (in my case, 3), the primary pattern, followed by the second most prolific tumor pattern found (in my case, 4), also known as the secondary pattern.

According to *Wikipedia* there are five patterns which reflect the known features of the tumor as follows ...

Pattern 1: The cancerous prostate closely resembles normal prostate tissue. The glands are small, well-formed, and closely packed. This corresponds to a well differentiated carcinoma.

Pattern 2: The tissue still has well-formed glands, but they are larger and have more tissue between them, implying that the stroma has increased. This also corresponds to a moderately differentiated carcinoma.

Pattern 3: The tissue still has recognizable glands, but the cells are darker. At high magnification, some of these cells have left the glands and are beginning to invade the surrounding tissue or having an infiltrative pattern. This corresponds to a moderately differentiated carcinoma.

Pattern 4: The tissue has few recognizable glands. Many cells are invading the surrounding tissue in neoplastic clumps. This corresponds to a poorly differentiated carcinoma.

Pattern 5: The tissue does not have any or only a few recognizable glands. There are often just sheets of cells throughout the surrounding tissue. This corresponds to an anaplastic carcinoma.

The Gleason Score ranges from 0 to 10, with 10 having the worst prognosis. For a Gleason Score of 7, a Gleason 4+3 is a more aggressive cancer than a Gleason 3+4. So what this told me was that four weeks ago (when I had the biopsy) my cancer was considered to be moderately aggressive.

I couldn't help but spend a few futile seconds wondering what the score would have been a year earlier when the idea of a biopsy was first mooted. Nor could I help but wonder what the score was going to be in two weeks time after I'd had my operation ... at least that was not a futile notion as whatever was removed would be subsequently analyzed.

•

It being Saturday, we could do nothing about the tests until at least Monday so we spent the rest of the afternoon finalizing our plans for getting to and staying in Rome. The only initial complication was how we were going to get to and from the station at Lamezia—virtually inaccessible by public transport from Santa Severina. I wouldn't be able to drive on the way back so there was no point in leaving the car at the station as we had done on other occasions.

Getting to and from Lamezia notwithstanding, by the time we opened the first bottle of wine that evening we had booked the train to Rome on Thursday June 20 and two nights at the York Hotel, about six hundred yards from Villa Salaria. (We had decided not to stay in the same bed & breakfast where we'd stayed when I had the biopsy because there was a long flight of steps from the gate up to the house; also the hotel was closer to the clinic.)

On the Saturday morning we would move in to the clinic and return to the York the following Wednesday and remain there until Dott. Cappa said we could leave, probably the following Sunday or Monday. When we had a sense of when I was going to be allowed to travel, we'd book the return train journey.

The first bottle of wine was already half gone when the doorbell rang. It was our friend Denise whom we'd invited to eat with us that evening ... I had been so convinced that we were going to be sharing good news with her.

In retrospect it was a good thing to have had her company that evening for, as ever, we laughed (and drank) a lot together and that was the perfect antidote to the rest of the day. It also gave us an opportunity to see how it felt to share such news with a third party for we knew that, in the days to come, we'd have to get used to that.

●

And I suppose, you'll want to know how I was feeling at this end of this unusual day? Apart from pleasantly inebriated, that is.

Well, as you will have already gathered, I'm quite pragmatic ... if something breaks, the only was to get it working properly is to fix it. Or you can leave it broken.

I might still be able to pee against a wall from two feet but I knew that if I didn't get rid of this cancer then my peeing-against-the-wall days could be short-lived.

I also wondered if I might have been able to avoid this situation had I not been so convinced that there was nothing wrong with me a year earlier ... but I also realized that to go down such a road was emotional folly.

Back then I had almost certainly made an error of judgement but I had to forget about that for I had to deal instead with what was actually happening to my body now and in this new situation. I was confident that I was in the hands of a remarkable man, a man whose fervent passion was to use his skills to make me (and others) better.

And I knew that was exactly what he would do and that, ere long, I would be able to hit that wall from at least three feet away.

•

My friend from England got back to me to tell me about the course of radiotherapy and hormone treatment he had undergone and to say that, in retrospect, he now wished his urologist had recommended surgery more forcefully. It felt good to have my instincts rubber-stamped, even by just one person.

Before the day was done, there were two other matters to deal with ...

I emailed my friends Tañia and Adam in Albuquerque whom I'd first met on my trip to America the previous November and who were planning a visit to Santa Severina that summer ... arriving on June 21. It was a reunion I had been looking forward to for many months but now knew it would not happen ... and I was more than crestfallen.

And, finally, I emailed my nephew, my dear friend and occasional traveling companion Neff, and told him that we wouldn't be able to make his wedding in London the following Saturday after all.

That was the hardest part of the day.

Ten challenging days

"I didn't really want them to open up my body, so I tried to see if a few other things would work."

Steve Jobs quoted in *Steve Jobs* by Walter Isaacson (Little, Brown 2011)

The above, spoken by Apple guru Steve Jobs—a person I had admired since I first used a Mac Classic back in the early nineties—is one of the saddest sentences in the English language. It is no exaggeration to say that the sentiment he expressed ultimately killed him.

Nobody likes their body being opened up but sometimes it is necessary in order to survive and what I was about to experience in the ten days *before* they opened up mine felt, at the time, infinitely worse than the prospect of the operation I was preparing for.

The problem was essentially a cultural one, it was not understanding the protocols of having to get all those tests done and not really having a clue where to start.

As it happened the following day, Sunday, we were invited to a family gathering by our friends, neighbors and landlords, Silvana Gerardi and Rafaelle Vizza. The occasion was the *cresima* (confirmation) of their son Francesco and we were going to meet up with everybody at a hotel in the coastal town of Le Castella.

This would be our first opportunity to tell Silvana and Rafaelle and the rest of our adopted family about my little local difficulty and at the same time ask Silvana if she'd water the plants on the balcony while we were out of town.

As we expected, Silvana and Rafaelle were very upset to hear our news and Rafaelle immediately offered to take us to the station at Lamezia but couldn't pick us up when we returned in early July as the family would all be attending a wedding in Rome.

Another family member, Silvana's brother Aurelio—who lives in the apartment above us—was also there and so, knowing that he worked in the pharmaceutical department at Crotone Hospital, I asked him about the tests. He told me to make a copy of the list and drop it in that evening.

Later, when he saw what was involved, he suggested I go to my doctor, Rocco, and get prescriptions for all five tests. In the meantime, he would see what he could find out on the following day at Crotone Hospital.

As Aurelio advised, on Monday I went to Roccabernarda to see my doctor, to bring Rocco up to speed with what was happening and to get prescriptions for the various tests. At the time, because there were several prescriptions to cover the long list of blood and urine tests, I didn't pick up that he'd missed two, the X-rays and the electrocardiogram. I also didn't pick up that tucked away in the list of blood tests there was actually one involving a urine sample.

The word 'tests' seems a bit wishy-washy for what lay ahead—they felt more like the Labours of Hercules. So, in the interests of giving an accurate impression, from now on I will refer to them as 'challenges'.

These were the challenges I had to overcome before we got to Rome:

The lengthy list of blood and urine test challenge

The full body scan (CAT scan), with contrast, challenge

The bone density scan challenge

The X-rays of the thorax challenge

The electrocardiogram challenge

We didn't see Aurelio till quite late that Monday evening as we'd been out for a pizza with Denise. When we met up later, he told me I had to be at Crotone Hospital at seven-thirty the following morning where he'd arranged for me to have the body (CAT) scan.

He didn't mention any of the other challenges so, not unreasonably, I assumed that I was just going to Crotone for the Cat scan. Aurelio, on the other hand, had other ideas and was going for the full set.

•

At this point I need to clarify something that only became apparent to Kay and I just before we finally left for Rome some ten days later—the penny took a long time to drop. What we missed was an essential part of the Calabrian psyche which, at one level we *did* know but, in the context of arranging these challenges, we completely missed initially.

All our experience told us that Calabrians are an open and generous people particularly with the likes of us, *straniere*, foreigners. They, more than most other Italians people, understand what it is like to be downtrodden and at the sharp end of economic hardship. So, everyone who became involved in assisting us achieve our five-challenge goal was bending over backwards to be helpful over and above what we were expecting and, instinctively, they built-in to everything they did, said or suggested an element of saving money, of spending as little as possible.

Quite simply, at the time, we did not appreciate this unspoken component so, in my descriptions of what actually happened, I will try and point out when and how, with the benefit of hindsight, we got it all wrong.

•

On Tuesday morning at the crack of dawn we duly presented ourselves at the surgical ward at Crotone Hospital with a bit of paper with a name on it. We had to find Aurelio's friend Salvatore who, it seemed, was going to arrange the CAT scan. The arrangement had all the hallmarks of someone doing someone a favor ... in this respect the lack of formal paperwork was a clue.

Introductions over, Salvatore showed me into a small side-room where a nurse took a blood sample. Moments later a female doctor came in and she and the nurse were chatting when I heard the name Neill mentioned. I asked the doctor if she was Neill Adams' wife—Neill was the Englishman who worked at Bios where I went for my blood tests. She was indeed Neill's wife, she was Dott.essa Michela Chiarello and later we talked for a while about her time working as a doctor in Edinburgh which is where, of course, she met her husband.

Salvatore then told me that they couldn't proceed with the scan until they had the results of my blood test and that would probably take about two hours. So, to kill some of the time, Kay and I walked into town for a coffee which is when I had what seemed like a good idea ... I'd walk over to the other side of town to Bios and have all those other blood tests on Dott. Cappa's list. What I hadn't picked up from the list is that I ought to have taken a urine sample with me.

The first realization of this came when the Osvaldo, who'd just taken half an armful of blood, looked at me questioningly and said, "Piss?"

He took my puzzled expression as a sign that he'd used the wrong word.

"It is called 'piss', isn't it?" he asked nervously.

Before breaking the news to Osvaldo that I hadn't brought any 'piss' with me, we had a short discussion on the various words you could use in English for urine. 'Piss', I suggested, was not the most common term in medical parlance but that he could be assured that everyone would know what he meant.

I then owned up to my lack of 'piss' that morning and offered to remedy that there and then but, no, it had to be a sample of the first 'piss' of the morning. I assured him that the following morning I'd bring him some 'piss' to analyze. From that day to this, he and I always refer to a urine sample as 'piss'.

Just before I left Bios I bumped into Neill Adams who already knew that I was having an operation the following week as he had just spoken to his wife at Crotone Hospital. The medical jungle drums were already at work.

So, by ten that morning I had completed almost one of the five challenges, the only thing lacking was some 'piss'. But I was pretty confident that when I returned to the hospital, challenge number two, the CAT scan would be done and dusted.

Back at Crotone Hospital we were still awaiting the pre-CAT scan blood test results when Aurelio and his wife Rosa turned up.

Until that moment I hadn't realized it was Aurelio's day off and that he'd come into Crotone with Rosa just to support us. Rosa's role was to keep Kay company while he and I started ticking off the challenges. One of these, all the blood tests, was next on his list and I had to explain to a bewildered Aurelio that I'd just had them done at Bios.

The language barrier was always a problem but it was the unspoken language and the cultural differences that were at play here. I never expected Aurelio to give up his time that day and he never told me that he would; nor, apart from the CAT scan, had he mentioned any of the other challenges. Yet, from his point of view, he couldn't understand why we'd paid good money to have the blood tests at Bios when he could have sorted it out at the hospital at a more modest rate which may even have been as low as zero.

Much of the above is an example of trying to work out in retrospect what was actually going on at the time, of realizing that Aurelio had taken on the responsibility of sorting it *all* out, even if he hadn't actually mentioned his plan to us.

It was a gloomy Salvatore who emerged from his office with the results of the earlier blood test. This showed that my creatine level was too high to have the CAT scan. Apparently I could have reduced this level by drinking several pints of water the evening before instead of, as in my case, almost the same amount of red wine.

But Aurelio was not daunted by this setback. Salvatore was a nurse, not a doctor, so all he would have to do was find a doctor who'd sanction me having a CAT scan with a slightly high creatine score. For twenty minutes the two of us scoured the corridors of Crotone Hospital in search of such a doctor but to no avail, rules were rules and there was not, after all, going to be any CAT scan for little old me that day.

So we headed instead for another department to find the man in charge of the bone-density scanner who, it turned out, was someone I actually knew. I'd met Dott. Antonio D'Antonio a few years earlier when the then mayor of Santa

Severina inaugurated a Slow Food project in the town.

After a few moments of the 'I'm-not-sure-how-I-can-possibly-fit-in-another-one' routine—a typical Italian response to such last-minute requests—my details were entered into the system and I was to return in an hour to have the first part of the treatment that would prepare me for the actual scan later in the day.

From here Aurelio frog-marched me to Cardiology where he hoped to hook up with Lucio, a heart surgeon from Santa Severina whom we both knew and whom Aurelio hoped would be able to sort out the electrocardiogram challenge. Unfortunately Lucio was on holiday for the week so Aurelio had to rely on his second favorite doctor in the department who started off with his version of the 'I'm-not-sure-how-I-can-possibly-fit-in-another-one' routine but, regardless, he found me a slot at eight-thirty on the following Tuesday.

We were on a roll and quickly headed for the about-to-close *Cassa*, the cashier's office, where I produced my prescription for the bone density scan and prepared to pay as, of course, I couldn't have the scan without the appropriate receipt. It was only then that I realized I'd left my wallet with Kay and Aurelio hadn't enough in his ... still the cashier was a friend and Aurelio promised he'd settle up later.

Aurelio and Rosa said goodbye just as I was called in to have the preparatory 'jab' for the bone density scan, the injection of a small amount of radio-active material. Later my entire body would be scanned by a gamma camera which was sensitive to the radiation emitted by the injected material.

After the injection I was told to go out and have lunch and drink lots of water, at least two or three pints, and then come back around four for the scan itself.

It was just before five in the afternoon when we finally left

Crotone Hospital. We'd been in and around the hospital for nearly ten hours and hadn't a single result to show for it. The blood and urine challenge was nearly completed (though I couldn't now take the 'piss' sample into Bios until Thursday because of the radio-active material in my bloodstream); the bone density scan was done (I'd get the results on the Friday); and the electrocardiogram had been booked for Tuesday. I still had to sort out the CAT scan and the X-rays.

When we got home we were totally exhausted, nevertheless the first thing I did was email Dott. Cappa to ask his advice about what I should do about the CAT scan ... was it the case, I wondered, that if my creatine score remained high, I might not be able to have the scan at all?

His response was quick and straight to the point—he suggested I go to the Casa di Cura Santa Rita, a private clinic in Cirò Marina, up the coast from Crotone, where he was pretty sure I could get everything sorted. I emailed them immediately and waited all-day Wednesday for a response. None came.

Of course if I'd called them I'd have had a quicker response but experience told me that dealing with such matters in writing leaves fewer opportunities for the linguistic and cultural complications I've already alluded to. If, for example, Aurelio and I had been communicating in writing, then I would have had a better grasp of what he was planning.

Rightly or wrongly, on the Tuesday I had picked up that, as far as his friend Salvatore was concerned, that was my first and last opportunity of having a CAT scan as a favor to Aurelio. And I was fine with that, I had always assumed that we would pay for all these challenges. Also I did not want to put Aurelio in any sort of awkward position with his colleagues.

●

First thing on Thursday we were on the road again as I rushed my first 'piss' of the morning to Bios for analysis; I was to pick up all the results the following morning.

On the way out of Crotone, Kay was not slow to pick up that we were heading north and not west towards Santa Severina. I told her we were going to Cirò Marina, to the Casa di Cura Santa Rita.

The two women who manned (if women can man) the reception area at the clinic were truly amazing. The more senior admitted that she hadn't checked her emails for a day or so, still we were there now so all was not lost. We explained the problem ... I needed a CAT scan, X-rays of my thorax as soon as possible. When 'as soon as possible' turned out to be that I needed the results by the following Wednesday at the latest (as were heading for Rome on the Thursday), there was a sharp intake of breath.

Still, this woman remained undaunted and called the woman in charge of that department who turned up in the office a few moments later. Not surprisingly, our unexpected arrival precipitated another 'I'm-not-sure-how-I-can-possibly-fit-in-another-one' moment but our new best friend would have none of it. If Dott. Manlio Cappa needed this before operating on me and, Dott. Cappa being a cousin of the clinic's founder Dott. Caparra, then it would be done.

The following day, Friday, I was to return at eleven for the pre-CAT blood test and the X-rays and then on Tuesday at nine I was to return for the CAT scan itself and to collect the X-rays. The CAT result would not be available till at least five on the Wednesday, the evening before we left for Rome.

I produced the prescription for the scan and paid up and

said I would bring the one for the X-rays (the one I didn't yet have as Rocco had forgotten to do it) when I came on Friday.

That afternoon I drove to Roccabernarda to see Rocco and get those two missing prescriptions. En route we had a coffee with out American friend Vicki who volunteered her teacher husband Pasquale to collect us at Lamezia when we returned from Rome. Another piece of the jigsaw in place.

So, by the end of Thursday almost everything was in place. The only outstanding problem was that the electrocardiogram in Crotone and the CAT scan in Cirò Marina were now scheduled for approximately the same time on the same day in towns forty-five minutes apart. I could not change the CAT scan so decided I'd pop in to the cardiology department at Crotone Hospital the following morning (when we were collecting the bone density scan results) to see if I could change the electrocardiogram to another time or day.

That evening, in anticipation of yet another pre-CAT scan blood test, I drank no wine but downed over three pints of water instead.

•

Friday was as busy as Thursday.

First stop was Bios for the blood and urine test results—one challenge finally completed.

Second stop was Crotone Hospital for the bone density results but they were not ready because of a computer malfunction so we could have to collect them the following Tuesday afternoon. I also managed to find the doctor who had created a minor fuss when Aurelio and I had made the electrocardiogram appointment for Tuesday and—surprise, surprise—he had absolutely no problem in bringing it forward a day to the Monday.

Third stop Santa Rita for the pre-CAT blood test and the X-rays. I produced the prescription for the X-rays and was asked where the one was for the blood test. My blank look said I didn't have one because I thought, as it was part of the CAT scan procedure, I didn't need one. There was great consternation and initially I got the impression that I couldn't possibly have the blood test without this bit of paper. But when the dust had settled it turned out that I didn't need one at all—but, if I had brought a prescription with me, I could have saved myself about €17 ($23 / £14). I paid up willingly before having my two X-rays, the results of which I could pick up on Tuesday when I came back for the CAT scan.

That day, I also met, for the first time, a particular Santa Rita nurse who, it seemed to me, was never without a smile ... I recall hoping she was going to be in charge when I had the CAT scan.

Getting closer but, by the end of that first week (four days to be precise), I had successfully completed one challenge and when I say 'completed' I mean I actually had the results in my hand.

•

The problem with not having had that prescription for the pre-CAT blood test is yet another example of people doing their utmost to help us save a few euro. On our first visit to Santa Rita, I had been given a specific list of what the blood test would be checking on and I only realized later that I was meant to give this list to my doctor so that he could write me out the appropriate prescription. Once again, not being conversant with the process had caused a minor local difficulty ... something else had got lost in translation.

By the weekend we were both very tired and my arms felt like the proverbial pin cushions. On the Saturday we tried to keep to ourselves and from time to time inevitably our thoughts wandered over to London and the wedding we were missing.

On the Sunday we had arranged to eat out with a few friends locally but, unknown to us, this 'last supper' had escalated into something much larger and we found ourselves surrounded by many well-meaning friends. It was just what we needed after such a tiring and unpredictable week.

Though we didn't know it at the time the second week was to be as gruelling, if not more so, than the first. By Wednesday we were actually looking forward to the blessed relief of Rome and the laparoscopic radical prostatectomy itself.

To put our travels into perspective, the journey from Santa Severina to Crotone Hospital was just short of twenty miles; from Santa Severina to Cirò Marina, thirty miles; and from Crotone to Cirò Marina, twenty-four miles. Not huge distances in themselves but not a single one of those miles was on anything other than a single carriageway road.

Experience told us that when, in Calabria, you have an appointment for something like an electrocardiogram at eight in the morning, the one thing that will not happen is that you arrive on time, have the test, get the results and then go.

Being from northern Europe—and therefore inclined to be punctual—we did indeed arrive at Crotone Hosptial a little before eight and headed straight for the cardiac ward where we'd made the original appointment from where we were redirected to a small waiting room off the main concourse.

(Because the appointment was so early in the morning and

the same time as the Cashier's Office opened, I had already given Aurelio the prescription and the cash so that he could pay up on my behalf and then bring the prescription to me emblazoned with its 'paid' stamp.)

We were not the first, the waiting room was full; there were two doors off the waiting room, the one at the far end half closed the other shut tight but with a small unmanned window-counter to its right. There were no signs to indicate whether I should go into any or none of the adjacent rooms or just wait to be summoned so, nothing ventured, nothing gained, I poked my head round the half open door at the end.

Got it first time ... this is where I was supposed to go and within a few moments my chest was hooked up to the electrocardiograph and a switch was thrown. Five minutes later I was back in the waiting room clutching a small piece of card with a number on it—eleven. So clearly there were ten others who had appointments at the same time or, more likely, ten others who knew the system better than we did and had got there early to jump the queue.

A few others came after us which brought the total number up to about sixteen. About half an hour later a white-coated man came to the window-counter next to the other door, opened it and called out a name; somebody got up and was shown through the door; the door was always locked behind them. Each person was inside for about ten minutes before another name was called ... we started to count, all the time wondering how long it would take to get to eleven.

Some new faces arrived in the waiting room and we were surprised to hear their names called out before they got to us. By our reckoning they must have been getting close to eleven.

We had now been waiting close on two hours when another man in a white coat came in and knocked the door; he was admitted and then, a quarter of an hour later, reappeared at the other door (behind which I had had the electrocardiogram) and called out: "Number one!"

All that time we had been watching he wrong door and the wrong queue; our queue was just starting and it took about forty-five minutes to get to number eleven.

The doctor we spoke to was amiable and confirmed that heart-wise I was in fine shape. Not unusually, he asked about how we had ended up in Calabria and why I needed the electrocardiogram and I told him about my pending operation. It turned out that he and Dott. Cappa had gone to medical school together and he asked to be remembered to him. Like so many others, he spoke of Dott. Cappa in the language of esteem and his last words were, "You're in the best possible hands."

Two challenges finally completed.

•

By Tuesday it was four ... I collected the X-ray results when we were at Santa Rita in the morning for the CAT scan and later in the afternoon I picked up the bone density scan results from Crotone Hospital. Both showed that, even at sixty-eight, I remained a fine figure of a man.

At Santa Rita, I also collected the blood test results, the Santa Rita equivalent of the ones that had denied me the CAT scan at Crotone Hospital. I quickly checked the creatine level and found it was almost the same as it had been the previous Tuesday in Crotone and yet here I was in the queue for a CAT scan.

All the others waiting seemed to be clutching bottles of water and so I asked my favorite nurse—who was in charge of the CAT scans that morning—whether I needed to drink lots of water. She said I should (I wondered how everyone else seemed to know this except me) and that she'd be giving me something else to drink forty minutes before the scan. That 'something else' was barium sulphate an oral suspension which is used for improving the quality of X-rays of the gastrointestinal system.

I downed the barium sulphate in the allotted time and was ushered in to take my place on the bed of the scanner which then took about fifteen minutes to scan my body. But I was having a CAT scan 'with contrast' which meant that I had to have the whole thing again but with a dye (a contrast material) which would be introduced into my body through a vein in the arm.

I'm not sure what happened next as I was still lying down and couldn't actually see my arm ... all I knew was my favorite nurse was trying to find an appropriate vein and then something went wrong. She kept saying "Blood-blood, blood-blood ..." and laughing nervously as she sought paper towels. Every time I tried to raise my had to take a look, she gently admonished me and said I was to lie flat. Whatever was going on didn't seem to panic anyone—at some point a doctor arrived to have a look—and soon everything was under control again as she decided, like so many before her, that my other arm might be more productive.

Sporting largish bandages on both arms, I rejoined Kay ... my last challenge almost completed; tomorrow at five, I would have the results.

This was the day I started taking the medications that Cappa had said I should have and, that evening, I also received an email from him to say that I should present myself at Villa Salaria at eight-thirty on Friday morning. He used the word *prelievo* which I thought meant that we would be having a pre-op parley and that I'd then hand over all my results. It wasn't until Friday morning that I found out what *prelievo* actually meant.

•

By Wednesday evening, the evening before we were to set off for Rome, the challenges were all over; I had competed all five and had all the results ready for what lay ahead in Rome.

On the advice of Kay, on our way back to Santa Severina I invested in a couple of pairs of loose, dark, lightweight trousers, the sort that wouldn't be too hot at a time of year when I would normally be wearing shorts and, more importantly, would successfully conceal a catheter bag.

Back home I realized how tired I was and how preoccupied I had been—we had both been—with these challenges. They had pushed us to the limits and, although we had found the medical culture and the language perplexing and confusing, we had emerged unscathed ... apart from my poor arms, that is.

And on the plus side, unlike, many others my age, I now knew that, apart from one small local difficulty, I was a pretty healthy specimen.

Over those ten days we scarcely had had time to think about the operation itself and I knew that when, finally, I was on that train to Rome, I would feel an amazing sense of relief.

It did occur to me that maybe that had been the point.

Rome

It was mid-afternoon when we arrived at Rome Termini where we caught the Metro to Conco d'Oro, about four miles north of the city centre; from here we walked the last mile to the York Hotel. It was a hot June day and we probably would have been wiser to have caught a cab.

After checking in, we had a rest before heading out to familiarize ourselves with the locality before heading for one of Rome's few Thai restaurants but one that happened to be within walking distance. This, we believed, was to be our last proper dinner together for a while as I suspected I would be fasting most of the following day. And, as it is almost impossible to find non-Italian cuisine in Calabria, we were particularly looking forward to something different.

The next morning, as per Dott. Cappa's email, we arrived

at Villa Salaria, no more than ten minutes walk away. It was strange to be back here again but it also felt familiar and that was something we both found valuable.

By nine Dott. Cappa had not showed and I was having second thoughts about the meaning of his message. By nine-fifteen I decided to see if it was still on my phone and when I eventually found it I went and showed it to the young woman on reception.

"Go to the nurses' station on the second floor", she said as she made a call to tell them to expect us. I immediately knew where we were going and I had a suspicion why.

The nurses' station was where I had had my blood pressure taken the time I almost fainted after the biopsy and my suspicion was that I was going to have yet another blood test.

I was right and, as ever, I left with so many plasters and bandages that it looked as if I'd just stepped out of a war zone ... I have to say that two of these were covering up wounds from previous encounters with needles in Crotone and Cirò Marina.

For the first time we met Suor'Anna, the ward sister in charge who was very impressed that I had turned up with a complete set of test results ... it was as if I was the first ever to do so. Perhaps I was. She told us she expected us back the following morning about seven-thirty when we'd be shown to the room which was to be our new home for the next few days. Everyone was incredibly helpful and friendly and there was also a discernible awareness that what we were experiencing was probably more difficult because we were clearly not Italian.

As we were about to leave we bumped into Dott. Cappa and I was able to check what, if anything, I could eat for the rest of the day. It turned out to be a fairly benign regime ... I could have a normal lunch but only something light in the evening. Between the two I was to start the laxative regime he'd told me about last time we met and which he'd since reinforced by email. He told me too that my operation would be the second of the day, probably starting around midday; the Romanian man he'd mentioned would be the first.

On the way back to the hotel we picked up a couple of sandwiches for the evening ... we had already decided we'd lunch in a small Italian restaurant, Fuoco e Farina, which we'd spotted the night before.

•

When we returned to the hotel the man on reception laughed when he saw the state of my arms ... he, more than anyone, knew what I was about to go through as I'd discovered that he had undergone a similar operation several years earlier.

This short sojourn at the York Hotel was the first period of relative calm we'd had since I was told about my prostate cancer. It was only a little over twenty-four hours since we'd left Calabria but it was a good time ... some might say it was the calm before the storm but I preferred to think of it as the calm before the beginning of the end.

After our surprise pasta lunch and my last (for the moment) few glasses of red wine, we returned to the York Hotel where, at two, I took my first two sachets of the super laxative that Dott. Cappa had prescribed. Over the next two hours I drank over four pints of water and then at four I took another two laxative sachets and the same amount of water all over again.

As, for most of my adult life I have always been on the constipated side of the evacuating spectrum, I knew this stuff was going to have to work really hard to make any difference.

It did ... and many visits to the bathroom later, the only thing I was evacuating seemed to be water itself.

Oh, I almost forgot, there was one other duty to be performed in preparation for the following day's festivities. I borrowed some of Kay's depilatory cream—the stuff women use to remove leg hair—as one of the other preparatory 'medications' Dott. Cappa assigned to me that Friday involved the removal of all body hair from the navel down.

In the process I learned something really important ... depilatory cream was not really meant for skin as sensitive as the scrotum. But Kay enjoyed the spectacle.

•

We had our light sandwich supper before settling down to watch a couple of DVDs. Experience had taught us that, in many smaller European hotels, the choice of tele-viewing was generally limited to endless game shows in the local language and one repetitive news channel in English ... so *we* always travelled with a small DVD player and a Scart cable. And, of course, we both had iPads to while away the time.

Later, as I sought the succor of sleep, I thought about Rome and the three other times I'd been here. In those previous visits—once on a day-trip by train from Arezzo, once on flying day-trip to visit the American Embassy and once for a biopsy—I had never really seen much of this city and I knew that this fourth visit was not going to change that.

I was also aware that, over the years, the original saying, 'See Naples and die', had somehow morphed into 'See Rome and die' ... I, on the other hand, was looking forward to returning to this unique city sometime soon to marvel at its rich and glorious heritage.

And, for the record, was I afraid? No.
Did I have fears? Of course I did.

Saturday, June 22

... laparoscopic surgery is as good at treating prostate cancer as open surgery. Men also lose less blood, have less pain, and spend less time in hospital. Most men also recover and go back to normal activities more quickly than with open radical prostatectomy surgery.

www.cancerresearchuk.org

We trundled our cases up the hill from the York Hotel to Villa Salaria; it was just coming up to seven-thirty in the morning.

Suor'Anna welcomed us and asked one of her colleagues to show us to our new home for the next few days. The room had two beds, one clearly meant for business and therefore for me; there was a wardrobe, a fridge, a television, a couple of chairs, an en suite bathroom and a door out to a spacious balcony that overlooked the gardens.

Suor'Anna had already confirmed that my operation would be the closing feature of the day and preparations would not begin till around midday.

While we were unpacking, a doctor, already dressed in scrubs, came in to glean some details of my medical history and whether or not I'd ever been anesthetized before; I resisted the temptation to say only by Italian game shows. He also produced a consent form for me to sign before confirming once again that my services would not be required for another four hours or so.

His suggestion that we should just relax proved a tad difficult but we had each other, our trusty iPads and a handy cafè-bar downstairs.

It was about ten-thirty when we got up from our table in the café-bar and went over to tell the young woman on reception that we were just popping out for a short walk. Before we had even got to the door she summoned us back ... she'd called upstairs to check that this was okay and Suor'Anna said we were not to leave ... I think she thought we might do a runner.

Just before midday, a nurse popped her head round the door and said I should get into my gown and get into bed. An hour later they came for me.

•

I recall being pushed into the elevator and coming out the other end into a sort of undefined no mans land.

I recall being brought back to my room, Kay looking anxiously on as I was hooked up to the bedside monitoring equipment.

And I recall how cold I felt.

I had been in surgery for over five hours (this was longer than anticipated because of a slight hitch that I found out about later), scantily clad in an environment where the temperature is kept deliberately low.

So, although I did not know at the time why my teeth were chattering, everyone around me did and soon my temperature got back to normal.

At first, although I was drifting in and out of sleep, I felt no pain. But gradually, as the effects of the anesthetic wore off I was aware of a fiery pain ... in both heels.

I was about to tell Kay about it when a nurse came in so I tried instead to get the message across to her without the Italian word for 'heel' in my vocabulary. I was pointing down the bed and wiggling my toes, still trying to get my message across to a nurse who thought I was pointing to my abdomen and who couldn't see my toes. I shook my head and then I had a brainwave ... the heel of Italy, of course, the heel of Italy is called Apuglia.

My remonstrations that Apuglia was painful fell on deaf ears so I shifted the focus to the part of Apuglia which was actually the heel of Italy, an area I knew well called *Il Salento*. When I started to say that *Il Salento* was really painful, the penny dropped with Kay and she was able to indicate the message I was trying to get across.

Then, of course, it became so obvious that everyone in the room couldn't believe they'd missed such a brilliant and imaginative description of *il tallone*, the heel. Still, we'd both learned a new word.

Apparently the reason for the painful heels was the fact that I'd spent so long at a slight angle on the operating table and my heels were taking much of the downward pressure from the weight of my body. And the remedy was simple, someone propped up my ankles with a pillow and the pain was gone.

I never felt any pain in my abdomen that evening or subsequently except when getting out of bed or out of a chair.

Dott. Cappa popped in to see how the Irish half of his international duo was faring. He told us—though Kay remembers more of the conversation than I do—that the operation had lasted longer than normal as they hit a slight snag when the catheter tube would not pass into the bladder as the rejoined urethra was too constricted. This had to be remedied to allow the catheter to pass through which added half an hour to the operation. Because of this extra surgery, I would have to keep the catheter in situ for three weeks (instead of a week to ten days) to give everything more time to heal.

Up to that point I was not aware of the catheter at all nor of the drain which exited my abdomen on the right side.

•

The nursing team that looked after me that first night were wonderful and coped steadfastly with my ebbs and flows. After the cold spell and the sore heels, I became incredibly hot and felt as if I was burning up. One of the nurses had a brainwave and fetched something that felt like a cold-bag which she placed on my abdomen ... Kay later told me that the nurse had 'borrowed' a pack of my blood from their fridge.

And later still, when Kay was wakened by an alarming sound from the machine that was monitoring my vital functions and the nursing team arrived on the scene, that blood came in handy again ... this time as was intended, as a transfusion; I was also given oxygen. It was my blood pressure that was the culprit as, once again, it had plummeted.

Apart from these minor hiccups I had a reasonable night and was looking forward to less excitement the next day.

Sunday

After a prostatectomy you will have a drip into a vein in
your arm, and a tube (catheter) to drain urine from your
bladder. You may have a small tube in the wound to drain
any excess fluid that is produced. This tube is usually
removed after a few days
www.macmillan.org.uk

Outside I could see that Sunday was a beautiful, sunny
summer's day in Rome.

I was relishing the light and the peace when the door burst
open and two nurses came in to check that I was still alive, to
remove my oxygen mask, to empty and replace my catheter
bag, to empty and replace my drain bag, to take my blood
pressure, to extract a pin-prick of blood from my finger (to
test blood-sugar / glycemia) ... it was six in the morning, the
beginning of a new day in hospitals and clinics worldwide.

As they were attaching a second bag of blood to my
bedside gantry, they were momentarily interrupted when the
team from the night shift came in to say goodbye and told
me they'd see me again on Tuesday. It was a kind gesture ...
maybe I'd unwittingly given them their first entertaining night
in weeks.

After the new shift had finished with me, I got out my iPhone and went to the two texts I'd already prepared—one in English and one in Italian which both said that everything had gone well and I was feeling fine—and started sending them to friends and family. I had remembered not to put any names in the 'to' field until after the operation as the last time I prepared such a text in advance I accidently sent it to Kay to tell her I'd landed safely in Chicago the day before I left to go there.

It was while I was having my first ever blanket bath that I asked if it would it be possible to get up and maybe sit in a chair or walk a little and was told that maybe 'later'. I had a similar response when I asked for something to eat. I didn't really know if my restless night was normal or not. If not, these the nurses were probably 'stalling' me for all the right reasons. I *was* really hungry and I did want to get up but, in truth, only because I had heard that it was good to get active again as soon as possible after such procedures ... I was actually happy enough staying in bed and reading through my return texts.

I was now sitting up and had had a look at my scars. Of course I couldn't see anything more than a few small band aids and one a bit larger, the latter I surmised is where my cancerous prostate gland finally saw the light of day. On the other side, the right, there was the drain and down the middle the catheter tube which, at its end appeared to be three-pronged before it snapped into a tube that in turn fed a bag clipped to the left side of the bed. I remember thinking, how the hell did they get that thing up there ... I was glad to have been asleep at the time.

Until that morning I never realized how heavy an iPad is. Hitherto I'd never thought of it but in that hospital bed it felt like a tonne ... or maybe, just maybe, I was a bit weaker physically than I felt in my head. It was when I mentioned this to Kay that she reminded me I had undergone a major operation and one that had lasted longer than was usual. Until that moment I had not really thought of it like that.

I had a doze while Kay went out to get some fresh air and something to eat and drink for although, in theory, my treatment at the clinic include all meals, she had to fend for herself. She had stocked up the fridge with this in mind but she also needed to get out of the building from time to time ... it did us both good.

My doze was interrupted by voices and I realized that Dott. Cappa had come to see me and I could see him reading my notes by the bottom of the bed. He asked me how I felt and I said I was fine, a little hungry perhaps. He said I could have something at lunchtime and when I asked about getting up he could see no problem and said he'd have a word with the nurses.

Another two doctors came in, one asked me if I could break wind; he used the polite Italian word for this which momentarily threw me as I was more conversant with the other one. I replied, "I'm part Irish and part Calabrian, I can *always* break wind."

The second doctor wanted to examine my lower legs and as he did so checked that I had had no problems with them (apart from the heels, that is); this was clearly a routine check on possible post-operative thrombosis issues.

That afternoon the six o'clock shift of nurses became the two o'clock shift of new faces who felt obliged to come round and check all my vital functions.

As yet no food—though I could drink water and was encouraged to drink oodles of the stuff—and still bedridden, I naturally felt obliged to mention both. There were positive noises but at first no direct action until Kay later went out to tell them that I was ravenous.

It was mid-afternoon when a kindly orderly came in with a bowl of soup. Perhaps 'soup' is too generous a word ... it was more like a bowl of warmish, watery, flecked stock with the smallest pasta imaginable swirling round the bottom of the bowl. But I loved it ... I did all but lick the bowl.

Throughout the day I dozed on and off, fantasized about food, checked the phone and watched on the iPad as the world went about its usual business. I had reminded a different nurse that I was keen to get up, if only to sit in a chair, but had become resigned to the fact that it was unlikely that I was going to set a foot out of bed that day.

Some time during the afternoon, I was disconnected from the machine that monitored my vital signs and I became more mobile, albeit within the confines of my bed. Nevertheless it was an indication that one stage of my recovery was past and new one was beginning.

In the early evening another bowl of lukewarm flecked broth appeared followed by some slightly stodgy meat and creamed potatoes ... as it happened, the type of potato I like least. My hesitation about even trying either was taken out of my hands when the door burst open and Suor'Anna rushed in, told me not to eat another bite, made the orderly take it away and asked if I was diabetic. I said I wasn't (not as far as I knew anyway) and she explained that the latest pin-prick test indicated that I might be.

It was then that I confessed about the banana I'd eaten earlier for I knew that this might have resulted in a 'false' reading. She was convinced and thereafter each time the finger-pricking police came in, I asked to see the number on the little digital window.

At ten o'clock the two o'clock shift went on their way and a new team of nurses did their round of checks and, like the others before them, they monitored and periodically changed the various liquids dripping into my arm from my bedside gantry.

That night I learned how it felt to have a full bag of urine, hanging by the bed ... I knew there was something not quite right and I guessed that all that excessive water intake had filled up the bag sooner than anticipated. Kay deserved her sleep as much as I did, so I pulled the 'help me, please' cord by my bed and a nurse appeared and replaced my bag ... Kay woke just as she was leaving the room.

Otherwise I had a better night and slept as well as is possible when you have one bag filling up on one side, a drain from the abdomen depositing a custard-like residue in another, while one arm is hooked up to a cocktail of painkillers and other medications.

Monday

Walking promotes the flow of oxygen throughout your body and maintains normal breathing function. It also strengthens your muscle tone. Gastrointestinal and urinary tract function are improved by walking. These body systems are slowed down after surgery. Walking also improves blood flow and speeds wound healing.
www.uwhealth.org

Once again I woke to the six o'clock round of checks and balances ... I was getting used to people poking around my body and I knew they had my interests at heart.

Dott. Cappa arrived around seven, after breakfast and before the nurses had got round to giving me my blanket bath. He asked if I'd been out of bed yet and I explained that, though I'd asked several times, nothing had actually happened. He wasn't best pleased and headed straight to the nurses' station from where I could hear raised voices.

What happened next was not entirely unexpected. Two admonished nurses strode purposefully in and asked Kay to wait outside, the normal procedure when they were about to give the patient a blanket bath. But today's bath was to be slightly different.

It was clear to me that one of the nurses was more rattled by Dott. Cappa's telling off than the other ... one was aware that I, the patient, was the innocent party in all this, the other I think saw me as an upstart. They proceeded to rearrange my tubing and hauled me upright to sit on the edge of the bed where they began to wash the upper part of my body and change my gown. One, the kinder one, noticed I had a few bed sores and treated these with a spray just before I was frog-marched clutching my two bags and wheeling the gantry to the chair by Kay's bed where the blanket bath was completed. Again I was aware that one was being more gentle with me than the other. Thereafter, when I needed any assistance with anything that was potentially uncomfortable or invasive, she was the one for me.

Well, it *was* what I wanted ... I *was* out of bed. The nurses had disappeared and Kay had clearly taken the hint and gone downstairs for a cup of coffee. I was struggling to get to my feet when Kay returned, surprised to find me not tucked up in bed.

I was having difficulty in getting out of the chair and Kay gave me a helping hand to finally get to my feet. She found a suitably deep carrier bag into which we put the two bags attached to me, the urine and the drain. I was more or less upright and ready to take my first unaided steps with my gantry pole to hold on to with my right hand and my carrier-bag of goodies in my left and my backside sticking out the gown. Nevertheless, a fine figure of a man.

I shuffled towards the balcony, then back to the door, then back to the balcony ... for the next five minutes this was the extent of my kingdom before I realized that I'd had enough and sank back into the welcoming arms of the chair.

I was exhausted but also exhilarated by those few brief moments of relative normality. I decided to rest a while before giving it another go. I wanted to try and get out of the chair unaided and was happy for Kay to go and indulge in a bit of retail therapy, particularly when one of her goals that day was to find me a new beard-trimmer as I'd forgotten to bring one with me and was feeling decidedly scruffy.

Left to my own devices and more rested, I tried again, unsuccessfully, to get out of the chair. It was then I realized that, smart as this chair was, its lines were not user-friendly when it came to the likes of post-operative me getting out of the thing. This was mainly because its seat sloped down towards the back and even for someone relatively fit it would have required additional effort to get upright. Hospital furniture designers/buyers, please note.

My favorite nurse popped her head round the door and I took advantage of her arm to get back on my feet once again and to do a few more circuits of the room. Worn out once again I eased myself back into my least favorite chair.

I was not coping well ... at least I had convinced myself that this was the case. And that next quarter of an hour sitting there, weary and unable to get to my feet, was my lowest moment. Lower than the trials and tribulations of the five challenges, lower than anything that had transpired during that first night. For a few fleeting moments I couldn't see myself ever walking normally again until I fast-forwarded in my mind's eye to catching the train back to Calabria in a week or so and knew that somehow, between then and now, it would all get better.

When Kay returned she found me slumped in the chair with my head in my hands. She helped me back to bed.

She also recalled something she had read on one of the online prostate cancer forums; it was something an unusually honest man said about how he felt post-surgery. There was a brief time, he said, when all he wanted to do was cry. *His* openness made *me* feel better.

•

Something else was happening that day for I was also having what are called bladder spasms, a painful urge to urinate which, in my case, was probably a result of my bladder getting used to having an intruder, the catheter balloon. (The so-called Foley catheter is retained in place by a small inflated balloon inside the bladder.) Although painful and uncomfortable at the time, these spasms soon passed.

•

For the first time I had lunch at the same time as everyone else and knew I was now an accepted part of the system when I was given a menu for that evening and the next day and asked to make my selection.

I had swung round with great difficulty to sit on the edge of the bed in order to eat off the trolley and at first couldn't work out why I found this manoeuvre so difficult. If I was to get in and out of bed by myself this was something I had to crack.

Lunch over I started to play with the bed and realized that the nurses liked the bed platform high so that they could work on me without straining their backs. On the other hand, when it was nearer the ground I could swing out easier and have the security of feeling my feet touch the floor. Thereafter there was a constant mechanical battle between the nurses and me as I kept lowering the bed and they kept raising it.

Later in the afternoon I decided it was time to do a little more walking but this time with a purpose ... it was time to feel more civilized, time to try out my newly-charged beard trimmer.

Kay wheeled the gantry round to the right side of the bed and with the platform at rock bottom, I got up with ease, my feet firmly fixed to the floor so that I could raise my body to the upright position. I did a few more laps of the room before heading to the bathroom.

Revitalized and feeling more like a human being, I thought it was time I stuck my head out the door to take a look at what was going on in the wider world. It was at this moment that a large man wearing shorts was walking past. He hesitated for a moment and held out his hand.

"You must be Dott. Cappa's other patient." he said in near perfect English, "I was hoping we'd meet. I'm Dan."

"Must go, my wife will be here in a minute."

And off he went, round the corner and presumably back to his bedroom. Dan, the Romanian, spoke English.

I was trying to work out how it was that Dan seemed to be so much more active than me. I could see that he was definitely a physically stronger specimen and, I guessed, he was probably eight or nine years younger than me ... *and* (I was now clutching at straws) he *did* have a head start, his operation was a good six hours earlier than mine *and* mine lasted longer.

It was good to have met him and I hoped we'd meet up again and swap stories about catheters and drains, about how we met Dott. Cappa and which nurse was the most *simpatica*.

Later Dott. Cappa dropped by and checked me over. He said I was doing fine and was pleased that, at long last, I'd been out and about. He'd also heard that Dan and I had met and explained that, though Dan was Romanian, he'd lived for many years in Italy, close to Rome, and that his wife and family were all Italian. I wondered where he'd learned his English.

I was just about to broach the subject of when I might leave the clinic when Dott. Cappa himself brought it up ... he thought I would be well enough to leave by Thursday but it could even be earlier, it depended on my progress. At the time, I just couldn't imagine it.

A little later another doctor popped in, a woman who just wanted to say hello as she too was from Calabria and had heard about us. Indeed she was from a part of Calabria which we knew well and where we'd once stayed with a friend.

So, although Monday had started off badly, it had ended better than I could have ever imagined during that one brief, dark moment when I was slumped in the chair with my head in my hands. In that moment I was close to tears and when I recall it, I well up with exactly the same emotions of complete hopelessness that I experienced then.

•

The urine bag that was emptied on a regular basis never actually contained anything that resembled urine; it *was* urine, but blood-red urine. This was normal. My bladder had to settle and get used to having a catheter there. I could expect it to clear in a day or two but for the moment blood-red it would be.

Once again during the night I had the same sensation that the catheter bag was full and needed emptying and replacing; this time I was able to partially get up and check for myself before calling for help.

The nurse who came to assist me decided that my bladder needed flushing out so, in order not to waken Kay, we crept to the bathroom where she inserted a liquid-filled syringe into the open end of the catheter tube, pushed the liquid into the bladder and then drew out a blood-red mix. She did this several times and I could that see long stringy clots were being exuded. It was a little uncomfortable but I could see for myself the good it was doing.

She fitted a new bag and I went back to bed, happy that this had all been accomplished without disturbing Kay ... *and* I had found another nurse that I liked. I made a special point of thanking her again the following morning.

Tuesday

Constipation is a common side effect of pain and bladder spasm medications. During the time that you are taking them, be sure to increase your fluid intake (at least eight glasses of water a day), take stool softeners, and eat lots of roughage (whole grains, fruit and vegetables). Use laxatives only as a last resort.

www.urology.ucsf

I was getting used to having my sleep interrupted by the early morning frenzy of checks and balances and was pleased to see that the new morning shift was the same team who had got me through that first night. They were like old friends.

Once again Dott. Cappa arrived around seven and before my blanket bath. He seemed happy with my continued progress and said he'd see me later.

As soon as breakfast and the blanket bath were out of the way I lowered the bed and got onto my feet with much more grace and confidence than I had the previous morning. I was walking better too and decided that, as and when I needed to have a break, I'd sit on the edge of the bed rather than the badly-designed chair. I still wasn't confident that I'd ever be able to get out of it unaided.

Kay was going down to the café-bar for some breakfast then out to do some shopping so I thought I'd clean myself up and maybe even wash my hair before going out for a walk in the corridor. That walk proved to be a major turning point for, no sooner had I stepped outside than I bumped into Dan and we walked and talked together for over an hour.

We swapped notes about all sorts of things and found that our prostate experiences, pre-Dott. Cappa, were not dissimilar in that we'd both seen other urologists and it seemed we'd even had our biopsies on the same day. We found too that we'd both had the same experience on Sunday when we'd kept asking to get up but nothing happened; Dan looked a bit sheepish when he explained how Suor'Anna had told him to calm down and to remember that he'd just had major surgery.

Above all we both felt that we had been incredibly fortunate to have met Dott. Manlio Cappa when we did; we agreed he was an extraordinary individual.

Dan was an extraordinary man too, a giant of a man in every sense. He was born and educated in Romania where he spent his formative years living under the harsh communist regime of Nicholai Ceausescu. Dan became a respected folk singer and, through his music, a dissident of sorts. He was not a political activist, rather someone who used his words and music to influence others. In April 1981 he finally left Romania and found work in Düsseldorf in Germany.

It was in 1987 that he came to Italy to work in IT where he settled and married his Italian wife, Stefania.

Dan's folk singing days are over but he is passing on his gift to his sons one of whom, it seems, is an accomplished guitarist while the other has a voice like his father.

And lately Dan has found unexpected fame through YouTube where one of his most famous songs—a song protesting about how the Ceausescu regime got rid of all

Romania's horses and replaced them with tractors—has been given a new lease of life with some clever graphics. Later we watched it together on my iPad.

We talked a little about his home country pre- and post-1989 when the Ceausescu regime was finally overthrown and he was surprised to hear that Kay and I had Romanian friends and had actually visited Romania the previous year.

As we walked and talked, we knew we'd both undergone a unique, defining experience. We were aware that this experience and this hour together had established a bond between us that would help us both through whatever these next days and weeks would bring. Independently we knew these things ... but it was all unspoken. We just knew it would be so.

And it was and still is.

I hadn't noticed that Kay had returned and slipped back into the room while Dan and I were out of sight. She told me later that she heard our voices and decided to leave us to our mens' talk; she could hear our laughing.

When we returned to our respective bedrooms—where I worked out that we had just walked about a thousand yards—I felt re-energized; if Dott. Cappa had come in at that moment and said I could go home, I could probably have done it.

It was just twenty-fours since my lowest point—my brief slumped-in-the-chair moment—to this, the highest. It was hard to believe that such a transformation was possible in such a short space of time.

I was buzzing and felt I needed to do something else to harness this feeling and felt slightly frustrated that nothing immediately came to mind. On reflection that was a good sign for it meant that I was beginning to think beyond the confines of my immediate environment. I decided I'd probably used enough physical and emotional energy for one day and settled instead for a pre-lunch nap.

I did some more walking later that afternoon, most notably when I took a card with my contact details round to Dan, lest we forgot. He gave me his and, like young star-struck lovers, we vowed to keep in touch.

When Dott. Cappa came round later he asked me if I'd been to the toilet yet, by which he meant had I voided, evacuated done number twos. The answer, of course, was no, I hadn't so, as this seemed an important part of the 'being discharged' process, he said I should take a spoonful of Levolac, a stool softener ... that would do the trick.

He sounded convincing but I knew that, at the best of times, my bowel movements generally responded to something more powerful than the usual over-the-counter medication. The stuff I'd had a few days earlier at the York Hotel was the only sort of thing that was going to guarantee explosive action.

But, as Dan had already told me that his spoonful of Levolac had done the trick, I went along with it and downed my spoonful and waited ... and waited ... and waited. As I suspected, nothing happened, scarcely a murmur.

It was getting late and I gave up waiting for the 'call to action' and went to sleep, safe in the knowledge that the only way I was going to shift the last three days' intake was with something a little more powerful.

Wednesday

Since you have a catheter your nurse will:
• show you how to look after it
• give you some spare overnight catheter bags
www.guysandstthomas.nhs.uk

On his early morning visit Dott. Cappa had unexpected news for me (and Dan too, I discovered later) ... if the current progress continued, then I could go home later that day; 'home' in our case would be the York Hotel. Almost in the same breath he asked me whether the Levolac had worked (as a bowel movement was part of the deal when it came to being discharged) and I had to explain that my system was a hard nut to crack and that I didn't think a stool softener was up to the task.

Dott. Cappa pointed out to me that it was important in the short term that such movements are made without any straining or pressure on the bladder so, as such a scenario was completely outside my normal experience, I suggested a sachet of the same stuff that had cleared me out the night before the operation. He agreed and a few moments later my favorite little nurse appeared with a sachet and advised me to stay close to the bathroom.

Before he left, Dott. Cappa gave Kay a list of medicines she was to buy that would help keep me infection-free and build up my strength over the next few weeks.

Kay took the opportunity of my preoccupation with bowel movements to go to the pharmacy after which she walked down to the York Hotel to confirm that we would be returning that evening. While she was gone I had countless false alarms and therefore lots of practice walking purposefully to and from the bathroom.

When Kay returned I still hadn't done the business but I *had* washed and dressed with real clothes including my baggy trousers. Just before lunch, when I'd almost given up hope, the deed was finally done—without strain, without pressure, like water from a sluice.

I was relieved beyond belief in every sense of the word.

By being involved in these extra-curricular activities that morning I was not unaware that I had managed to avoid another blanket bath. It was no coincidence ... I had deliberately decided that I would be more gentle with my bits than someone who didn't know what it was like to have bits ... especially bits with a tube up the middle.

Besides, I needed the practice ... if I were to be discharged that evening then I needed to know how to keep myself clean and infection-free. With regard to the latter, Suor'Anna had earlier told Kay about a particular anti-bacterial liquid soap for 'intimate hygiene' which we were already stock-piling. We had also invested in some disposable, pre-soaped washing gloves. There was no doubt I was going to be the cleanest guy in town.

During the afternoon we started to pack ... or rather I looked on as Kay packed. It seemed incredible that exactly a week earlier we had been at the Santa Rita clinic in Cirò

Marina collecting the CAT-scan result and now here we were preparing to move into the York Hotel for the second time in six days. Two days earlier I could not have foreseen such a transformation.

At two that afternoon the nursing team had changed and the new shift was the same team that had gotten me through that first night ... to me it felt fitting that I should leave Villa Salaria on their watch.

There were certain formalities to go through. For example hitherto I had never changed a catheter bag, I had watched others do it but after today this would be something I would have to get used to doing myself. Also, I knew there were two types of bag—the larger-capacity overnight one, the only one I had used thus far, and the smaller strap-to-the-thigh version which I knew existed but had never even seen. The latter was for normal, everyday use and generally would be inconspicuous underneath my trousers.

First I was shown the technique for disconnecting and connecting, then advised that I always do it over a toilet bowl as there was no way of controlling what dribbled out between disconnecting one bag and attaching the next. I was also told that at no point should any part of either the catheter or the bag itself come in contact with the toilet bowl. Hygiene around the whole changing operation was of the utmost importance.

Then I was shown how to attach the smaller bag to my thigh and given some narrow lint bandage with which to do this. It was clear this technique was a get-you-home Heath Robinson way of doing things and I had no confidence that it would work in the long-term without restricting the blood flow to my lower leg. But at least it would get me to the York Hotel.

We were also given a small supply of both types of bag—it

was recommended that I change the smaller one every day and the overnight one every couple of nights—and a protective sheet for my side of the bed in case of accidents.

Before I was finally fitted with the new, petite version, my bladder was once again flushed out and slowly, miraculously, what had been blood-red moments early began to change to a color more associated with urine, a sort of blush color.

So now that the tubing that I was used to carrying on my left-hand side was sorted out, all that remained was for the tubing on the other side—the drain—to be removed.

Dott. Cappa arrived about seven and checked that I had finally done the 'other' business and was good to go.

I was ushered onto the bed and he, assisted by the Polish nurse who had used my pack of blood so inventively a few days earlier, removed the stitch holding the drain and then the drain itself. It was all over in a flash and seemed as simple as it was pain-free.

Dott. Cappa checked that I had everything I needed for the next few days, particularly my medications, and said he wanted to see me on Friday morning to check and probably remove my stitches and to see that all was fine. He expected I would be fit to travel on the following Monday after a final check back at Villa Salaria late on Sunday.

As far as Villa Salaria was concerned, I was now free to go.

Well, almost free ... there followed many emotional farewells which started—and finished—with Dan who, like me, was preparing to leave. Together, like veterans of some long-remembered wartime campaign, we did the rounds of the second floor of Villa Salaria and thanked everyone for their many kindnesses to each and to all of us. Back at the nurses' station we embraced Suor'Anna and her team of nurses and orderlies and our Calabrian doctor friend. In the background there appeared a face I didn't initially recognize until his hand shot out from the group to shake mine ... it was the duty doctor who had looked after me that Saturday afternoon, what seemed a lifetime ago, when I had to return to the clinic following my post-biopsy dizzy spell.

Dan was waiting for a friend to collect him and carry his bags and so we said our final good-byes by the elevator and promised to keep in touch via email and phone. I looked up at him and said we should do this Italian-style so we two non-Italians embraced, hugged and kissed twice; for both of us it was a special moment.

Down at reception Kay called a cab and ten minutes later we were settling in to our temporary 'home' in the York Hotel.

I felt both elated and a little nervous.

The York Hotel

Make sure the [catheter] bag is always lower than your bladder. This keeps urine from flowing back into your bladder.

www.nlm.nih.gov

While Kay went out in search of food, I set up the DVD player before arranging the bathroom so that everything I might need during the night was to hand. I also gave some thought to how I was going to keep the catheter bag upright through the night. At Villa Salaria, the bag itself hooked onto a clip attached to the side of the bed but I knew that was not going to work here.

There was, I assumed, a reason why the bag was always kept upright at the clinic ... perhaps if it were lying flat on the floor the neck could become restricted where it formed a right angle with the tube coming down from the bed. I noticed that the box containing the soap-impregnated gloves was tall and narrow, exactly the right shape, so I started with that (the gloves themselves were individually wrapped). It was perfect except that I could see that, if there were sudden movement once the bag started to fill up, the box would have a tendency to fall over and in so doing defeat the object.

I was still trying to resolve this when Kay returned and we tucked into a late lukewarm dinner from the local supermarket.

While we was eating I noticed my sandals sitting by the bed and wondered if the base of the 'catheter' box would wedge firmly enough between the two straps to keep it vertical. I checked later and it did ... I had created the perfect night-time way of keeping the catheter bag lower that my abdomen and in an upright position.

Later, before going to bed, I took forty-five minutes to complete my ablutions, including my first ever changing of the catheter bag. I was scrupulously hygienic and incredibly gentle on the parts of me that I thought might be sensitive, particularly where the catheter tube emerged. I was trying to establish some sort of routine in the knowledge that I would be doing this at least twice every day, morning and evening.

During the night I again had the sensation that my bag was full—and it was. So I took what seemed an age to get out of bed without disturbing Kay and get myself to the bathroom to empty it, a process that I was soon to become used to and more adept at performing quickly.

•

Next morning I cut my time in the bathroom down to forty minutes and re-emerged with the smaller daytime catheter bag insecurely strapped to my upper thigh.

At the York there was no elevator from the ground floor to the lower-ground where the breakfast room was located so we had to use the stairs. This felt much better than I had been expecting ... I just had to take it easy on the way back up. Still, we were in no rush and it was all part of my self-inflicted mobility regime.

The catheter bag I was finding awkward, not per se, but because it felt insecure and had already slid down my leg during breakfast and was therefore all but hanging on the tube emerging from my penis.

In my head I knew the solution but imagined that we could not get hold of the necessary components until we returned to Calabria. So instead I began looking for alternative methods to keep the bag from taking on a life of its own and wandering around my thigh willy-nilly.

I made several attempts at suspending it from the belt line of my trousers but this proved just as awkward because it had to pass beneath my boxer shorts. I tried fixing it to the waistband of the boxers themselves but, as it began to fill, the weight began to pull the boxers down. I came up with a truly Heath Robinson device made with a 'chain' of safety pins which an unconvinced Kay went out and bought for me.

She returned with an assortment of safety pins and I set to work enthusiastically to solve the catheter-bag conundrum. She had been right, the safety pin idea was useless.

For the remainder of that day I put up with the inconvenience of the less-than-perfect roll of lint from Villa Salaria and gradually got better at making the bag stay in the one place for longer. Nevertheless it *always* slipped down eventually.

The weather was typical for late June in Rome—gloriously sunny and warm—and so we spent some time sitting out on the balcony or walking in the garden at the back of the hotel. I was feeling confident that I was truly on the mend and could feel myself getting stronger and stronger. Even my urine was a better color.

That first afternoon I decided to have a short nap and lay on the bed for about an hour. When I got up I felt a little odd and noticed that the urine in the 'daytime' bag still strapped to my left thigh had become decidedly bloody.

It took me only a few moments to work out what had happened: because I had been lying more or less horizontal on the bed with the bag still attached to my leg, the urine had nowhere to go and, in addition, some from the bag had almost certainly returned to my bladder. If I felt like an afternoon nap in future, then I would have to change to the larger 'night-time' bag with the longer tube ... or doze in a chair.

It was a salutary lesson and yet so obvious and a mistake I never made again.

I was still cutting back on the ablution time in the bathroom and that evening felt good when I finally dropped off.

Nevertheless I still woke up with what I thought was another full bag, the sensation of needing to urinate was the same as the other times when the bag was full. I slowly got out of bed and, carrying the box containing the bag, headed for the bathroom. Here I found that the bag was not completely full but that there appeared to be some sort of obstruction in the tube. I'd seen this before in the clinic and knew it to be a stringy clotting of blood, a thin six-inch long clot working its way down the tube at its own pace and therefore restricting the normal flow of urine (over which, at the time, I had no control).

I decided to help it on its way by disconnecting the bag, upending it over the toilet bowl and forcing it back up the tube and out—apart from the pressure I used on this occasion, this was how I normally emptied the bag. It worked but when I went to reconnect the tube to the catheter, I noticed another stringy mess on its way out. I wasn't sure if I should just watch it until it eventually came out or whether I should help it on its way by pulling it. I opted for the former but grew impatient and resorted to the latter.

I slowly helped it on its way down the tube and out and the urine flow then continued normally. Having washed my hands and both catheter connections, I reattached the tube to the catheter. I was just about to return to bed when I noticed, at the top of the catheter tube itself another clot was starting its painfully slow progress southwards and I knew I'd have to wait till it stuck its nose out before I could help it on its way.

By the time Kay woke I'd been up just over an hour. By the time I finally got back into bed, reasonably confident that stringy-clot-man up there in my bladder had given up for the night, I'd been up almost three hours.

I couldn't be sure why this happened but I suspected that it was not unconnected with the fact that, earlier in the day, I'd let the urine that was already in the catheter bag drain back into my bladder.

I knew that such clotting was not unusual and I was not worried about it, I was just frustrated that it had kept me up for so long ... particularly as, the next morning, we had to be up early to return to Villa Salaria for the first of my two check-ups before I could go home.

•

The following morning, Friday, as I lay on Dott. Cappa's gurney while he removed my stitches—more like metal staples—I told him about my de-clotting shenanigans earlier that same morning. He didn't seem perturbed and said he would scan my bladder and check for clots.

The last staple-stitch gone, he covered each wound with a tiny band-aid so that the skin could breathe and then did the bladder scan. We both looked at it on the monitor—though, in truth, I had no idea what I was looking for—and he said it all seemed fine and was clot-free. He wasn't concerned that my urine was still quite bloody and said this was normal.

He told me I would have the catheter removed on July

13 at Crotone and gave me a packet of ten man-size diapers which he said I would need for some time after the catheter came out—I would certainly need them for a week or so, a few months even, there was no way of telling; everyone was different. He suggested I would regain control of my bladder more quickly if I were to do some Kegel (pelvic floor) exercises which strengthen muscles below the bladder that in turn help control urination.

At my instigation we talked again about the biopsy, I was curious about what he'd said about the samples not travelling well at thirty thousand feet. He told me how he used to do the biopsies at Crotone and then brought the samples back to Rome for analysis (at that time there was a direct flight between the two cities). He repeated that he felt they underwent some change during the transportation process that may have had an impact on the veracity of the result.

He told me how a greater problem arose when, for security reasons, he was unable to carry them with him on board and they had to go in the plane's hold. On two occasions the airline lost the bag containing the samples and the poor patients had to have a second biopsy.

It was then he decided to drive to and from Crotone and that he would only do biopsies in Rome.

Finally, I told him that we had come to the clinic by taxi (six hundred yards uphill) but said I wanted to walk back to the hotel if he thought that was a reasonable activity at this stage in my recovery.

He said it was ... and I did.

Before we left, I arranged to see him again late afternoon on the Sunday. He was going to be in Crotone that weekend and suggested that if I hadn't heard from him by four, then I should text him to confirm when he'd be back in Rome.

On the way back to the hotel, we stopped off at the pharmacy around the corner, the pharmacy where Kay was now a regular and almost on first-name terms with one of the assistants. We were there to buy the first month's supply of Chalis, the form of Viagra that I was to start taking that weekend ... I have to say there was a heavy intake of breath from both of us when we heard the price!

I asked about the smaller, daytime catheter bags and was shown a pack of ten in which I could see what looked like some sort of flexible strap which was clearly designed for the purpose of holding the bags in place. The bag I was wearing at that very moment was already wandering around my thigh even though I'd emptied and readjusted it before leaving the clinic.

We knew sooner or later we'd need to buy some more of these smaller bags so we bought a couple of packs.

Back at the York Hotel, I felt exhilarated by the walk from the clinic and enthused by the prospect of having some sort of made-for-purpose straps holding my catheter bag in place.

At this point I should explain that each bag has, in each corner, a reinforced vertical slit (less than an inch in length) through which the straps (or lint, or whatever) pass. As most people's upper legs become narrower between thigh and knee, then the tendency is for anything that is not elastic or flexible to wander downwards and in so doing to put the short flexible link between catheter and bag under some pressure.

I therefore assumed that these white rubber straps—punctuated with small holes like a watch-strap—would do the trick. I felt so confident about them and my walking ability that, just before lunch, we went out for a short stroll to the small café a couple of hundred yards *uphill* from the hotel.

We sat outside in the sun and had an ice-cream, safe in the knowledge that my catheter bag was fixed securely in place.

And it was ... except that when we got back to the hotel I noticed that one of the straps had disappeared completely and the other looked as if it was about to break where the holes were. Although I had four such straps, I knew there was no way they were going to get me through the next two weeks.

I explained to Kay that the only thing that would work efficiently was wide piece of elastic cut to the appropriate length with a two-inch overlap with velcro stitched to both ends. And where were going anything like that on a Saturday afternoon in a quiet suburb of Rome?

The frustrating thing about all this was that, had I not had that complication at the end of the surgery, then that Sunday Dott. Cappa would probably have taken out the catheter. As it stood, I would continue like this for another fortnight.

So I was resigned to the fact that we'd get it all sorted when we got back home. Nevertheless, later that afternoon, Kay went out on a mission and returned with a yard of wide elastic, two strips of velcro and a needle and white thread. An hour later I was strutting round the room in my underpants showing off my new, made-to-measure catheter-bag straps. They were perfect ... they never shifted, never restricted the blood flow to my lower leg and never broke. I still have them.

That evening I spent less than half an hour in the bathroom before climbing in to bed. I was looking forward to a clot-free night though, as expected, I did have to get up once to empty my bag. Apart from that, I had a normal night's sleep.

•

Contact with the outside world was maintained via our iPads through which we received and sent messages, watched the daily news, played games and generally whiled away the time. We even played Scrabble against each other on our iPads.

I had noticed that there were bus-stops either side of the road close to the hotel and had taken a mental note of the three route numbers that Saturday morning on our walk up to the café ... I was interested because I had come across a neat little iPad app called Moovit which gives details and timetables of public transport almost everywhere in the world. I was of course interested in Rome and in particular the bus services that ran along Via Cavriglia.

I had two motives for this new interest in bus timetables for Kay and I had both had enough of the lukewarm dinners we had eaten for three evenings. Don't get me wrong, we were both appreciative that there actually was a local supermarket that sold such things but the time was right for a change ... and a change meant going further afield.

I had a plan. That evening we would walk to the Italian restaurant, Fuoco e Farina, where we'd had lunch the day before my operation. That was certainly doable, it was downhill and we were in no rush. Afterwards we'd catch the bus back up the hill to the hotel provided we could trust the timetable.

Now, if that worked on the Saturday and I got the 'all clear' from Dott. Cappa on the Sunday, then we'd catch another bus that evening and eat once more at the Thai restaurant, Isola Puket, where we'd eaten a week earlier. Depending on how I felt, we could catch the bus back again or get a cab.

So Saturday afternoon found us sitting on the easy chairs close to the hotel's reception desk ostensibly playing on our iPads but all the time I had one eye on the passing traffic and in particular the buses that passed and *when* they passed.

Moovit's timetable was spot-on ... all the buses, in both directions, came and went when they were supposed to. And later, when once again we were sitting outside our favorite café having an ice-cream, I was able to predict with amazing accuracy which bus was about to pass and when.

We were about to embark on a new chapter.

We left the York Hotel just after half-six to walk down to Fuoco e Farina. We were in no rush and surmised that the walk, punctuated with a bit of window-shopping, would take us no more than half an hour.

In rural Calabria, and most other parts of southern Italy, people eat no earlier than eight in the evening so, not surprisingly, restaurants rarely open before then. This being the big city we expected it to be different (we had found it so in other parts of Italy) so we were more than a little surprised to find that Fuoco e Farina didn't open till seven-thirty.

I didn't feel like walking and standing for an additional half-hour so we sat outside at one of the restaurant's sidewalk tables and waited. Not surprisingly we were the first customers of the evening.

It is hard to describe how wonderful it felt to be doing something completely normal like eating out. It was just over eight days since we had eaten at this very table but it seemed a lifetime ago since I had done something so ordinary. I was scarcely aware that I had a bag strapped to my thigh for I was confident that when I returned to the York Hotel it would still be there ... a little fuller perhaps, but still there.

And then, sated and paid up, we walked round the corner to the bus-stop and a few moments later caught the bus 'home'.

It was such a good feeling.

•

Off and on throughout Sunday we spent some time organizing our luggage for the following morning when we expected to finally leave the York Hotel and head by cab back to the station, Roma Termini. I was so confident that Dott. Cappa would sign me off that afternoon that I had already booked our tickets back to Lamezia Terme online and the hotel receptionist had printed them out for me.

In the warmth of the morning we walked to the café for our usual mid-morning coffee. It being Sunday there were more people about and the Sunday-morning newspaper-reading habit was, I noticed, universal. I remember thinking that I was almost certainly the only person at that moment who was peeing into a bag beneath the table. I noticed also that the number 92 went by, right on schedule.

Back at the hotel we decided who was going to carry what between cab and train: Kay would take both cases and, in addition to my iPad, I would carry a couple of lighter carriers which mostly held my medicines, spare catheter bags and related sundries.

As four approached I texted Dott. Cappa but did not get an immediate response. When I did, it was to say that he was behind schedule and that he had arranged for his colleague, Dott. Valentini, to see me at Villa Salaria at five. Dott. Valentini was the doctor who had assisted Dott. Cappa with my biopsy.

I had already decided that I was fit enough to walk up to Villa Salaria ... it took just five minutes longer than the first time we'd walked there pre-surgery. Kay was not impressed when I suggested I might run back afterwards ... as it happened that would have been totally out of the question.

Dott. Valentini checked my wounds, cleaned them and re-covered them; he also cleaned round the catheter. He then said he would need to flush out my bladder as my urine still showed no signs of recapturing the alluring blushing yellow hue it had had earlier in the week. This he did a little more vigorously than others had done but it was very effective for soon the urine coming out was more like it should have been.

He put me back together again (by which I mean he reattached the catheter) and of course was duly impressed by the innovative, already-patented leg-strapping apparatus.

He said I was free to go—to go back to the hotel and to go back to Calabria.

An hour-and-a-half later, Kay and I were standing on Via Cavriglia waiting for the number 92 to take us to Isola Puket. It arrived on schedule and there followed a bare-knuckle ride courtesy of a maniacal driver which, on more than one occasion, nearly threw me out of my seat. If ever there was a test for my poor bladder and its sundry attachments, it was this. Everything survived the experience but I was so keen to get off that damn bus that we did so a stop too early and had to walk further than expected to get to the restaurant.

But it was worth it for we both enjoy Thai food and it's something we never get the chance to experience in Calabria. It was a fitting end to our time in Rome ... not surprisingly we returned to the hotel by cab rather than catch the bus. The cab driver, eager to emulate, my earlier experience on the bus chose a route back to the hotel that included several roads that were cobbled which had much the same effect as the bus.

•

It was Monday July 1. After breakfast we said farewell to all our friends at the York Hotel. Their generosity to Kay and their concern for me had been over and above the call of duty and for that we were grateful. I had already written and uploaded my Trip Advisor review—next time we were in

Rome we knew exactly where we'd stay.

At the appointed hour the cab pulled up outside and we headed through the Monday morning traffic to the city center and Roma Termini.

We soon found what we thought was the correct platform only to find that, twenty minutes before departure, this was changed to another as far away as was possible from where we were waiting. Kay rushed on ahead to get to the train and find our seats and I trundled along behind as fast as I could; I knew we had plenty of time.

The last thing I had done before leaving the hotel was empty my catheter bag and I expected to have to empty it again at least twice on the five-hour journey to our destination, Lamezia Terme.

The journey itself was tiring but otherwise uneventful. I focused on arriving at the other end with a just-emptied catheter bag, of seeing a familiar face (Vicki's husband Pasquale) on the platform at Lamezia and being driven home to Santa Severina.

More than anything I was looking forward to sleeping in my own bed.

Santa Severina

Do not do any heavy lifting—anything more than 10 to 20
pounds—or strenuous exercise for three weeks following
surgery. You can increase your exercise schedule gradually
thereafter. Driving is usually permitted after the catheter is
removed if you feel comfortable.
www.ucsfhealth.org

On the platform at Lamezia, Pasquale told me that I looked
really well. I'm not sure what he was expecting but, whatever
it was he saw, it did seem to genuinely surprise him; in fact he
mentioned it several times.

On reflection I think what he saw, what I couldn't disguise,
was my pleasure at being back home, being back in Calabria,
being where I wanted to be.

I was happy and it was clearly written all over me.

Pasquale dropped us off as close to our home as is possible
and he and Kay carried the suitcases down the short slope to
the house while I made my own way down at a more leisurely
pace. Once inside, the first thing I did was empty the bag I'd
been slowly filling on the hour and a half drive home.

Kay went round the house opening all the shutters on both

floors to let the bright Calabrian light back into our lives. It was another good moment in this day of good moments ... like when the train pulled out of Rome station; like when we ran alongside the Tyrrhenian Sea south of Sapri and the short-lived Basilicata became Calabria; like when we saw the beaming Pasquale on the platform at Lamezia; and like when we turned the corner out of San Mauro and saw Santa Severina atop its hill just a few miles across the valley.

That first evening we were getting used once more to the Calabrian heat; we were also on a high from just being back here atop this small hill. It was half-ten, it was hot and we needed some exercise so we went out for a walk.

We strolled along the narrow road that links our side of the town with the outside world. There were others, mostly women and children, sitting outside their homes seeking a breath of wind and some cooler air before going to bed. We ran the gauntlet of people wondering where we'd been these past few days, of others in the know who wanted to be assured that everything had gone well, of one who asked me why I wasn't walking as fast as usual.

Finally we were past all the houses and in a brief no mans land where we could look out across the valley to the lights of the other small towns scattered across distant hills. You could almost feel the silence and touch the heat.

It was now a week since I sat in my room in Rome with my head in my hands ... back then I could not have imagined being here like this.

Slowly we walked back home, fielding a few more questions and many good wishes from those for whom it was still too hot for bed.

Monday was assuredly a day of good moments but the most precious was when, after only twenty minutes in the bathroom, I fell into bed and let my overnight catheter bag hang loose in its new, sturdier, sandal-less box.

•

Normally it's a five-minute walk from our house up to the town square. In this case the word 'up' does actually mean upwards, in the sense of a climb. There was no getting round it ... to get to the town's square you have to climb.

It was Tuesday morning and Kay was going to do some basic shopping down at the small supermarket in the lower town, a twenty-minute walk down, nearer to half an hour back.

Kay had her doubts, but I persuaded her that we should meet in the square; she would text me when she left the supermarket, I would estimate how long it would take both of us to make it to the square and hopefully we would meet en route, or in the square itself.

Kay wasn't sure I should try to walk all the way up there so soon after getting back but I knew I could make it, I *wanted* to make it. And I did—I took it slowly, stopped a few times to regain my strength and to admire the view and we met more or less where we expected our paths might cross.

Our immediate goal was Carlo's bar but, as soon as we entered the square, all those who knew where we'd been came to greet us, to hug and to kiss us and to welcome us back to Santa Severina. It was an emotional morning and it was fitting that we should bump into both Franco Severini and Dott. Rizza.

It was the first of many such occasions that week as we were reunited with friends in and around the town. The next day I walked up and back twice.

We were of course confined here as Kay didn't drive and I couldn't while I still had the catheter. I found the best way to explain the catheter usually involved one or more of the following: to offer to show it to people; to make light of it; to make it a normal part of my healing process; to say how convenient it was not to have to go to the bathroom. At no point did I ever feel embarrassed about it.

Yes, we were confined to the town but Santa Severina is a good place to be confined for, every day, there are the little three-wheeled utility vehicles that are common in Mediterranean countries as well as more normal-sized vans that visit every part of the town selling fruit, vegetables, fish, cheese, bread and cooked meats. For all of these the furthest we had to walk was fifty yards.

People who dropped in had different expectations as to how they would find me. Some clearly expected that I would be sitting back in a chair with my feet up in front of the television; one was surprised to find me in the kitchen, access to which is via a spiral staircase which he thought I couldn't possibly negotiate; another—who had known I was to have surgery—didn't realize I'd already had it and asked when I was leaving for Rome.

Apart from not being able to drive, in terms of our day-to-day routines, it was ostensibly business as usual. I had managed to cut down my twice-daily ablutions to no more than ten to fifteen minutes, was managing to vacate regularly —and without over-exerting—with the help of a hefty daily dose of Levolax, aided and abetted by prunes in yogurt; and my urine retained its healthy color. Around the house I was doing all the things I was used to doing—cooking, working at my computer, making bread.

Of course, I did have one or two 'accidents' when I failed to plug my bag in properly but these were few and far between and of little consequence ... and, of course, my own fault. Generally I could feel myself gaining strength and almost every day was able to do something I couldn't do the day before: like open certain shutters (which required a pulling action on a strap) or carrying fruit and vegetables home from the van at the top of the street.

•

I was scheduled to have the catheter removed on Saturday July 13 in Crotone so I had to work out how to get there as public transport was infrequent to say the least. I asked our friend Carlo about his nephew, Gaspere, and wondered whether he would drive us in our car that morning for a small financial consideration.

The arrangement was made—Gaspare would meet us by the car park at nine-fifteen which would give us plenty of time to get to Crotone to see Michele (Dott. Cappa's nurse) at ten as arranged. I had built in a fifteen-minute buffer to allow for the fact that southern Italians are rarely on time for anything. In most cases, five or ten minutes late was considered acceptable.

At nine-twenty-five a call to Gaspare's mother ensured that we were finally on the road by just after nine-thirty-five. We arrived at Dott. Cappa's surgery three minutes late, something generally unheard of when *we* are in control of events; Michele was waiting for us.

We had come equipped with a diaper from the pack that Dott. Cappa had given us in Rome; at home we had already received delivery of an additional sixty that we had ordered on the internet. I knew that the next few weeks, months even, could not be predicted with any certainty. In terms of urinary control, some people get back to normal quite quickly, others can take up to a year or longer. The Kegel (pelvic floor) exercises are meant to help with this and although I had done these before going to Rome and since too, I had lacked the discipline to get on top of the recommended three-time-a-day routine.

I knew that Dan (who'd already been without a catheter for over a week) was finding life in diaper-land very frustrating and was becoming impatient with the process, with always being on the lookout for the nearest restroom. I recall sending him what I thought was an encouraging email saying that he shouldn't worry and that it was normal for it to take a few weeks or a few months, even longer. His frustrated reply reminded me that he was now past the few weeks stage.

So, for the first time I didn't know what was around the corner, how easy or difficult it was going to be for me to learn to urinate again with some sort of control.

But I hadn't got there yet. I was sitting apprehensively on Michele's gurney, holding on to my drawn-up knees, watching Michele fiddle with the little screw-knobs on the side of the catheter which, I assumed, was how he deflated the balloon inside my bladder. It goes without saying that, though I was looking forward to my body being a catheter-free zone, I was not really looking forward to the process of having the catheter removed.

It was over in seconds and was no different to having the drain removed before I left the clinic in Rome; I was aware of something passing through me that made me want to purse my lips but that was all; painful or uncomfortable it was not.

Ten minutes later, and sporting my first diaper, we were back in the car with Gaspare and heading home. But not empty-handed—I had persuaded Michele to give me a souvenir of these last few weeks. I wanted to keep my catheter; I wasn't sure what I was going to do with it, but I wanted to keep it.

We went straight to the town square where I could share the news with everyone, the news that I was catheter-free and could drive. It felt really good and though I could urinate freely into the diapers any time I wanted, I still tried to recognize the signs and go to the bathroom.

That evening we went out to eat; we went by car.

Post-catheter

A bladder spasm is a contraction of the bladder which generates an urge to urinate, sometimes accompanied by extreme pain. Incontinence may occur if the bladder spasm continues, as the contraction will force urine out.
www.en.wikipedia.org

I felt so good that first evening that what happened next was both unexpected, debilitating and painful. Also, what I experienced was neither unusual or commonplace, it was just something that happens to some and not to others.

From Sunday to Tuesday I had bladder spasms; I had some respite on Wednesday, more spasms Thursday until on Friday I was spasm-free ... and remained so thereafter.

Just as my bladder had reacted to the arrival of the catheter, it now seemed to be reacting to its withdrawal. Unlike Dan and others who have the same surgery, my bladder played host to the catheter for three weeks. From trying initially to reject it, it got used to it and now it had to get used to its removal.

On Sunday the spasms crept up on me; once every hour became once every half-hour, every fifteen minutes even. I would have the sensation of wanting to urinate with scarcely enough time to get to the bathroom and lower my trousers. Sometimes I would actually urinate, other times no more than a trickle. I had no way of knowing which it would be.

Trickle or normal flow, the end result was the same— excruciating pain, why-me pain, repeated-expletive pain, fist-banging-against-the-wall pain. And then, half a minute later, it was all gone ... until the next time.

The nights were the worst for, since returning from Rome, I had got used once again to the wonderful normality of sleep only to have it snatched from my grasp. The first night I woke up ten times; the second night (Monday-Tuesday) fourteen times. Each visit to the bathroom was the same, the same sense of despair and the same pain.

The following night was better and Wednesday itself was a good day and I thought I was over the worst. But the spasms returned for one final foray on Thursday, albeit less frequent and less painful. And by Friday they were gone.

I had gone through so many diapers that week that I ordered another sixty for I could not be sure what was going to happen next. I actually only ever saturated one diaper (and that was the first night), the others were rendered redundant by either not being able to get it off quick enough when I had a spasm or no more than a dribble here, a splurge there.

Because of the spasms I'd not yet really had the opportunity to learn to control my bladder but as soon as I realized the spasms were gone for good, that became my priority. In the bathroom I would practice starting to urinate, then stopping, then starting again until, after a relatively short time, I became quite good at it. A bit like old times.

The 'splurges' I had that resulted in a diaper change were generally when I made sudden movements, laughed or passed wind. Most people would, I suspect, have added sneezing to that list ... as would I had it not been for my dentist in Croatia. Because of the work he did for me in March—and in particular the sinus lifts—he had taught me how to control a sneeze as I had to avoid sneezing for at least two months following the sinus work. So, by chance, the fact that I could control the urge to sneeze was a great help in keeping more of those little splurges at bay.

Within a week I was using one diaper a day and one at night and most were discarded for no more than hygiene reasons.

●

Monday July 22 was a special day. Not only was it a month since I'd had my operation but it was the day I would go to Crotone for the first of three monthly blood tests to check my PSA. The ideal number was, of course, zero. On the following Saturday I was to see Dott. Cappa in Crotone to tell him the result of the PSA test, some other tests he asked me to have and to hear from him the histological analysis of what he removed.

On Wednesday we drove back to Crotone for the results; my PSA was 0.08 ... almost as near to zero as you can get. We were more than delighted; and again the next day when we heard that Dan's was 0.07.

The appointment with Dott. Cappa started off as a light-hearted affair. He was pleased that the PSA was what he expected and he said that the histology report suggested that I needed no further treatment. The cancer had been removed.

He went on to show us the pathology analysis which indicated that, in the five weeks between biopsy and surgery, the cancer had become more aggressive—on the Gleason scale it had gone from 3-4 to 4-3, in other words pattern 4 was now more dominant than 3. The report also indicated that the cancer was at stage three (in a scale of four) and therefore that we had been fortunate to have acted when we did.

As we drove back to Santa Severina, I wondered what might have happened had we gone instead for surgery in late July which, at the time I had the biopsy results, had been the other option. Indeed, consideration of that scenario remained with me for some time afterwards for I realized two things.

I now knew beyond doubt that I had made an error of judgement back in the spring of 2012 when I found out that my PSA was on the high side. I should have been more pro-active and swayed less by how I felt.

I also knew that I had been incredibly fortunate. The information we now had indicated that the cancer was on the ascendency and that, had I waited until July, there might have been a different prognosis.

Later I wrote to Dott. Cappa to thank him once again. I also explained that I didn't fully understand the protocol of such things in Italy but that the last time I saw him I had to resist the temptation to give him a great big hug. I'm sure he understood how I felt and what I was trying to say.

•

The long, hot Calabria summer got longer and hotter.

On the Monday after I saw Dott. Cappa I stopped wearing diapers during the day; it was the same day another sixty arrived that I'd ordered when I was having the bladder spasms.

I continued to wear one every night for about a week but then discontinued these too. Instead I wore a little 'leakage' pad stuck to the inside of my boxers. Generally these remained dry all day and all night ... the biggest problems remained sudden movements, laughing and passing wind though the latter I was more able to control.

July became August and every day I felt stronger and stronger; the memories, good and bad, began to fade. As far as I was concerned I was back to normal and even the Cialis was beginning to work.

I was writing again too. *Thank you Uncle Sam*, the book that I'd researched in the United States the previous November and had been working on in the spring with a view to finishing that summer, was now back on course. I was hoping it could be finally published in October.

On August 12, a few days before that peculiarly Italian mid-summer festival known as Ferragosto, we picked up our friend Ivano at Lamezia Airport—for me the longest drive (about and hour and a half each way) I had done in several months.

Though he lived in England, Ivano, more than anyone, was responsible for the fact that Kay and I ended up living in Italy. We had met up in the UK a few times since we'd made the move but this was the first time Ivano (a fluent Italian-speaker) had been to Calabria. It is hardly surprisingly therefore that we had a propensity to burn the candle at both ends.

There was a lot happening that week in and around Santa Severina and on two successive nights we didn't get to bed until three in the morning. Between the two we also drove into the Sila mountains to spend some time with Vicki and Pasquale and their family.

It was a wonderful feeling that finally things had got back to normal and that, at long last, I was not taking any drugs that interfered with my predilection to enjoy Calabrian wine.

All too soon it was Friday and time to take Ivano back to Lamezia and send him on his way.

As Kay and drove back to Santa Severina, tired but still buzzing after the marvellous time we'd had with our dear friend, we had no idea that those few days had taken their toll on me. We had no idea that my immune system was not yet back to its robust self and the indulgences of those few days were, for it, the last straw.

We had no idea that our summer had just ended.

Later that day, I realized I had succumbed to what the Italians call *il fuoco di Sant'Antonio*, literally 'the fire of Saint Anthony'.

Il fuoco di Sant'Antonio ...

... is an infection of a nerve area caused by the varicella-
zoster virus. It causes pain and a rash along a band of skin
supplied by the affected nerve. Pain sometimes persists
after the rash has gone, more commonly in people over the
age of fifty.
www.patient.co.uk.

Il fuoco di Sant'Antonio is herpes zoster or shingles to
most people.

In the early eighties I'd had a mild dose of shingles around
one half of my body, from chest to back; but this was
decidedly different. This time it homed in on where I was
most vulnerable, on where I'd had my surgery ... the penis,
the scrotum, the perineum and adjacent areas.

It was not a good time ... and the worst thing about it was,
it was almost certainly self-inflicted.

After a false start with a local doctor (whom I visited only
because my doctor, Rocco, was on vacation), it was clear I
had shingles. Both Kay and I recognized the rash and this was
confirmed by many photographs on the internet. I was not
using the internet as a means of diagnosis, rather a means of

affirming what I already knew. And, as ever with the internet, there was conflicting advice as to what I could or should do about it.

So I turned to the one person who'd had recent experience of that part of my body ... I emailed Dott. Cappa. He got back to me within half an hour to tell me what to get and how long to use it—I was to administer an antiviral cream, take an antiviral tablet, both for five days, and take Vitamin C for a couple of weeks.

Apart from the fact that it put my complete recovery from the prostate surgery back several weeks *and* it was probably self-inflicted, it was a thoroughly unpleasant episode—sitting was painful, standing uncomfortable and lying down just about bearable. The fact that it was painful to sit had a knock-on effect in that it set the book I was working on back still further. I also had to reschedule my final dental visit to Croatia until I was one hundred percent fit.

So, although by mid-August, eight weeks post-surgery, I felt completely fit, my immune system had remained fragile and, unwittingly, I paid the price. It was almost another six weeks, around the end of September, before I felt I was back to where I had been in mid-August. It was a salutary lesson, hard-learned.

•

As I write it is just over six months since my surgery and I feel as fit as the proverbial fiddle.

In October I finally went to Croatia to have my last dental treatment and I now have a smile to die for. On my return I stopped wearing those stick-on anti-leakage pads ... in my boxers, that is, not on my teeth.

My PSA score has remained at zero; from now until next summer I will check it at three-monthly intervals and thereafter twice a year. I suspect my friends at Bios are happy to be seeing less of me.

The three-month Cialis program has successfully completed its work and everything in the erectile function department is fine. And for those who are desperate to know the nitty-gritty of how an orgasm feels without ejaculate ... well, its eye-rollingly good, possibly stronger than before and definitely less messy.

And yes, all those stories you've heard about the penis being shorter than before are true ... but, hey, I'm half Irish, half Calabrian, I can live with six Irish inches, fifteen Calabrian centimetres. Or is it the other way round?

Other side effects?

Well, this is difficult to assess for it is all to easy to attribute a natural change to a specific event, or to the wrong specific event. So the 'changes' I have noticed are not necessarily the result of the cancer and my subsequent treatment.

But they *could* be.

Kay tells me I smell different. I am sometimes aware of this when it is extremely hot—which of course happens a lot here, even in the autumn—when I seem to exude a more 'aromatic' perspiration that previously.

My previous position as a life-long stalwart of the irregular/constipated—the Italian word is *stitico*, a word I prefer as it has a more onomatopoetic ring to it—wing of the evacuating spectrum has shifted somewhat and I seem to have taken up more of a central position, still veering occasionally towards my old forsaken habits but definitely more regular and consistent (in both senses).

And related to the above ... when I feel I have to go, then I have to go. Previously I could put it off for an indeterminate length of time but those days have passed (pun intended).

I do not take any other drugs except my daily tablet for high blood pressure.

Finally, in mid-November, I finished *Thank you Uncle Sam*. I had already started to write this book.

Looking back ... looking forward

Writing this book was never part of my plan. This time last year I had absolutely no idea that there was anything cancerous lurking in my body. All the signs to the contrary I either ignored or rationalized into something they weren't.

So this is the philosophical bit ...

My general good health and the fact that I have always watched my diet and my weight—and can still run faster than many men twenty-five years my junior—gave me a false sense of my own vulnerability.

For too long I ignored the one sign that said something *might* be wrong because I was aware of its inconsistencies as an accurate indicator that something was indeed wrong. And for that error in judgement—which I would like to think was uncharacteristic—I almost paid too high a price.

I have thought long and hard about why it was I did this, why I allowed myself to be hoodwinked into creating a cosy little cocoon for myself that was a cancer-free zone.

Like Steve Jobs, I do not like people poking about my body ... but then I don't really know anyone who does. I have always considered myself a medical coward and generally have feared the anticipated pain of any such procedures. And yet I voluntarily opted to have invasive and extreme dental treatment which, my wife Kay has told me, she could *never* have undergone.

I generally have faith in the medical profession, both their professionalism and their skill. I know that sometimes things can go wrong and, when that happens, it is the nature of the job they do that the consequences can be more serious.

It is also the nature of the media to focus on the one failing and ignore the millions of normal procedures that have a predictable and unsensational outcome. It is so much easier to criticize a perceived error than it is to commend the routine and the ordinary ... if it were not so then we wouldn't have the tabloid press.

In the light of what I have just written, it would seem clear that I had no reason to fear a biopsy, either the procedure itself or the outcome. Yet when this was initially suggested back in the spring of 2012, I backed off, I didn't have it done.

I realize, of course, that there is now no point in pursuing this line of thought any further—even with the benefit of hindsight, I cannot come up with any reasonable explanations, just a hotch-potch of random possibilities which may or may not have contributed to my thought processes at the time.

The only important thing is that I finally got off my backside and did *something* and, it would appear, just in time.

•

I did however think back to that first meeting with the urologist in Roccabernarda and try to understand better what was happening. You may recall that he gave me a list of five things—chocolate, spicy meats, chillies, beer and coffee—that

I was not to consume. Neither at the time nor subsequently had I ever wondered why these foods in particular. I expected that there was evidence to show that they could result in a high PSA score which in turn could be an indication of an inflamed prostate gland or something worse.

So, a bit late in the day, I thought I'd see what I could find out and chose my favorite, chillies, *pepperoncini* as it's called here. I searched on the internet for *piccante e cancro della prostata* (*piccante* is the general term for hot, spicy foods, including chillies). I then did the same searches with coffee, chocolate and beer.

With the caveats I have already alluded to regarding such searches and the media's interpretation of them, I found that all of these foodstuffs were generally supposed to be good for prostate health, a term which generally refers to the prevention or alleviation of benign prostatic hyperplasia rather than prostate cancer.

Not surprisingly some sites went over the top in the language they used to extol the benefits of each and one claim from 2009 caught my eye which said that eating chillies caused eighty percent of prostate cancer cells to 'commit suicide'. If only the ones lurking in my prostate gland had read that article, I thought.

I didn't find anything that explained to me how (or even if) any of these might have affected my PSA score and so was still at a loss as to why, if they were generally good for me, I had to eliminate them from my diet.

•

I realize that I have put my urologist, Dott. Manlio Cappa, up there on some sort of pedestal. I have thought long and hard about this too, after all, is he not just a doctor who is simply doing his job? The answer is, of course, yes, but how many doctors or consultants do you know who regularly make a thirteen-hour round trip to give back something to the community where he or she was raised? Not many, I suspect.

So, even before I met Dott. Cappa, I already knew some things about him. I knew that he was respected among his peers and throughout the Italian peninsula and I knew too that he had a side to him that revered and remembered his roots. He had a humanity and I knew I would like this man.

I remember too sitting in the reception area at Villa Salaria the day of my biopsy. Kay and I were people watching and in particular we were picking out the doctors as they came and went—they had a way of carrying themselves that exuded something different to the other mortals going about their business that morning. Suffice to say, Dott. Manlio Cappa was not like these other doctors.

And I recall when Dan Chebac told me about the time he first saw Dott. Cappa, initially relating to a kidney problem. Up until then Dan had had regular digital prostate examinations and PSA tests through his work, the most recent of which indicated that all was fine. But, shortly afterwards when Dott. Cappa gave him the same digital examination, Dott. Cappa picked up that something was not right and told Dan to have another PSA test ... and of course Dan's story ended the same way as mine.

But, at the time, Dan was keen to know how it was that Dott. Cappa had picked up on a potential problem when another urologist clearly hadn't; Dott. Cappa's reply was a single word, *artigiano*. This is the English word 'artisan' and I believe it was his way of saying that there are—as there are in every walk of life—those for whom their work is a job and there are those who eat and breathe their chosen calling. As an ex-teacher, I know exactly what he meant; at that time I was used to observing the same distinction on a daily basis.

Of course I realize there are other urologists who could have done for me what Dott. Cappa did but I suspect not all would have received from me, the patient, the same degree of trust, respect and confidence. I was fortunate, I didn't just *think* I was going to get better, I *knew* it to be an absolute certainty.

Our friend Denise, who ate with us on the day I found out I had prostate cancer, relived that evening in an email to me. She recalled how she realized that she was the most scared person in the room and that she marvelled at how strong Kay and I appeared to be. But her most vivid memory was of Kay telling her that she should feel very confident for we were in the best possible hands and that very soon I was going to be fine.

The difference between Denise's fear and our apparent ability to remain calm was that we had met Dott. Cappa and she had not.

•

When people ask me about this experience, the one thing they often allude to is their own variant of the question, "Was it painful?". Of course the short, trite answer should be "No", for everything around such procedures in hospitals and clinics is geared to making it as comfortable and pain-free as possible.

Pain and the anticipation of it are a strange phenomena. Depending on a person's previous experiences of pain, he or she will feel it in different ways and to different degrees; they will display different levels of tolerance.

When my father finally described to me what he went

through during the Battle of the Somme in 1916, I could not imagine the pain he must have endured, particularly during an operation without anaesthetic to save his badly injured leg. He in turn could not understand why, as my dentist, I was averse to him injecting me in the mouth.

What people *do* generally have in common is an inability to recall exactly what it was like at the time; pain is of the moment. Also pain itself includes a broad spectrum of sensations, from a feeling of discomfort to excruciating agony; likewise those who endure a similar level of pain will describe it differently. And intertwined with all these different shades, how do you evaluate pre- and post-pain bravado?

There is also the question of choice. I cannot imagine the pain of giving birth but for many women it is something they choose to endure; likewise, I chose to endure any pain associated with the dental treatment I underwent. I wonder is it easier to accommodate pain and the anticipation of pain if you are the one in control of events?

In retrospect my answer to Dott. Cappa's question about my dental treatment, which he asked while he was performing the biopsy, was truthful ... in 2013 the worst pain I felt was for a few brief moments in the dental chair in Croatia when the local anaesthetic was beginning to wear off. At the time Dott. Cappa asked me about this, I couldn't be sure. But now I am.

So here is my considered response to the 'pain' question ...

The worst pain I felt relating to my prostate treatment was the series of bladder spasms I had which started the day after the catheter was removed when I was back home in Calabria. My experience was, I understand, extreme and related to the fact that I had to use a catheter for a longer period than normal.

The worst emotional pain was the Monday after the surgery when I realized I couldn't get out of that damn chair unaided. I suspect that, post-surgery, many people experience a similar moment or phase.

The greatest prolonged pain and discomfort I felt was when I went down with *il fuoco di Sant'Antonio*—a much more descriptive label than 'shingles'. This was both a physical and a despairing pain, the latter because I knew it was my own fault and at the time I had been within a whisker of being back to normal.

●

All of that is in the past. What of the future?

Well, of course there are two futures to consider: there is the future of medical research and resulting prevention and detection techniques and treatments in the area of prostate cancer; then there is little old me.

Detection and treatment techniques will clearly move on and some of what I have described in this book may soon be obsolete. How and when this happens will depend on a combination of medical and technological breakthroughs and lateral thinking. It usually does.

Some of these different techniques are already filtering through and in some countries the MRI (magnetic resonance imaging) scan is already being used as a second line of defence after a first-time negative biopsy.

Detection techniques *will* get better: inevitably other screening techniques will come along that either complement and refine the PSA test or even replace it and, as early detection becomes more precise, so this will inevitably impact on treatments. Perhaps the treatment I had will eventually become a rare exception ... who knows?

All of this will be science-led; it will be doctors and scientists who, through their painstaking research, embracement and adaptation of new technologies, experience, innovation and intuition will ultimately make the difference to the prostate health of subsequent generations. My three sons included.

And when that happens, the pushers of 'breakthrough potions and miracle cures' will inevitably move on to something else, they will home in on another imprecise medical science to make (and take) their money and run.

And as far as 'little old me' is concerned, whatever the future brings health-wise, it will have nothing to do with the fickle finger of fate ... as I've already indicated I believe in fate as much as I believe in the tooth fairy.

At this moment in time I continue to be in the same good health that I thought I was in when I had cancer. So, unless I detect some symptoms to the contrary, I will assume that, at this moment in time, my body remains a cancer-free temple.

If there is to be a next time, then I believe that I will be more aware of it at the time. I think this experience has nudged me into giving more time to assessing how I actually feel before saying, "I feel fine". It's not something I'm preoccupied with, it's just a subtle shift in my thought processes.

Should I ever think there is something not right I will get it checked.

And if, subsequently, I have to add to my knowledge or need any sort of additional information or advice, I might well resort to the internet but I will not do so alone ... I will always have my trusty bullshit-button at the ready ...

Afterword

As I write this it happens to be December 31, the end of another year.

As you might expect, I don't really believe in numbers (PSA and Gleason scores excluded) in the sense that, had I had my first PSA test and my surgery on the same day a year apart, that would have been no more than coincidence. The numbers would be irrelevant.

So the only reason I mention that it is December 31 is that, as we do every year, Kay and I will celebrate Capodanno (New Year) with our neighbors and friends, the Gerardi family, and afterwards we will all dance to the music of the late, great Rino Gaetano.

Six months ago I would not have been able to dance.

Three months ago I probably could have danced but may have also had a 'splurge' or three.

Tonight I will dance because I can.

As ever, there will be a point in the evening when everyone will hug and kiss everyone else and say "Buon anno". Not long afterwards, as I do every year, I will subtly disengage from the group and, glass in hand, walk to the edge of the garden and look across the valley of the river Neto to the other hillside towns and villages sharing their firework displays with us.

For a moment I will think about this lofty place that I like so much and acknowledge how fortunate I am to live here and to have friends here. I will think about those who are special to me, many of whom, my wife Kay and the Gerardi family, will be only a few yards away.

I will shed an unseen tear.

Last year, when I did the same, I had no idea what lay ahead. This evening, when I take in the same view, surrounded by the same people, and have the same thoughts ... I still will have no idea what lies ahead.

But I will be a little wiser.

Niall Allsop ...

... was born and educated in Belfast, Northern Ireland, but began his working life as a primary school teacher in London and in 1971 took up his first headship.

He left teaching in 1981 to pursue a career as a freelance photo-journalist specializing in the UK's inland waterways and wrote extensively in this field both as a contributor to several national magazines and later as author of a number of related titles, one of which, in a fourth edition, remains in print.

By the early 1990s he was a graphic designer and the in-house designer for an international photographic publishing house in Manchester before becoming a freelance graphic designer based in the south-west of England.

In September 2008 he and his wife, Kay, moved to Calabria, the toe of Italy, where they enjoy a sort of retirement and where they continue to struggle daily with the language in a small hilltop town where they are the only English-speaking people.

Since moving to Calabria he has written several books with Italian themes and also a memoir relating to his teaching career.

Other titles by Niall Allsop

Thank you Uncle Sam
Calabrian Families in America

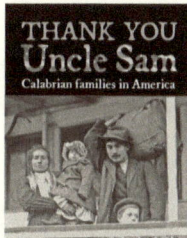

It has been estimated that twenty million Italians emigrated in the hundred years between the 1860s and the 1960s. The majority of these went to start a new life in the United States of America and of these by far the majority left behind family and friends in southern Italy.

From within southern Italy it was individuals and families from Calabria and Sicily—the areas of the most endemic poverty and perennial economic hardship—who formed the bulk of those who emigrated around the turn of the new century.

Post-war, in the fifties and sixties, America once again drew many from these same areas of deprivation, people for whom the post-war boom was something that was happening elsewhere.

As a resident of Calabria, Niall Allsop had met people who talked of family members in America, some of whom had emigrated as far back as the early twentieth century. Then, in the square of Santa Severina one summer, he met Gino Sculco from New Jersey who was enjoying a vacation back in the town of his birth. Gino explained how his father had emigrated in 1920, returned to Calabria and emigrated again in 1960, the second time accompanied by one of his sons. In 1967 Gino and his wife Sina followed in their footsteps.

Niall Allsop was so intrigued by the Sculco family's story that he decided to travel to America to find out more about what motivated them and other Calabrian families to emigrate. He was also curious to find out what happened once they got there.

Thank you, Uncle Sam is the result of that curiosity.

Stumbling through Italy
Tales of Tuscany, Sicily, Sardinia, Apulia, Calabria and places in-between

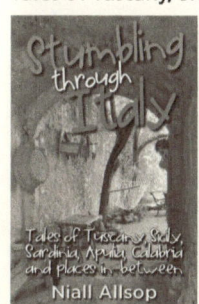

In September 1999 Niall Allsop and his wife Kay flew to Pisa and stepped onto Italian soil for the first time.

Within six months they returned and thereafter they visited Italy at least twice a year, usually to the most southerly provinces of Apulia and Calabria and the islands of Sicily and Sardinia.

They knew they holidayed differently to other people and in Italy, despite the lack of language, they found themselves somehow drawn into people's lives and homes; they had experiences and encounters that seemed to pass others by.

Stumbling through Italy is the prequel to *Scratching the Toe of Italy* and is the irreverent chronicle of their Italian travels and the many remarkable and colorful people they met there up to the summer of 2008 ... when, finally reconciled to the inevitable, they returned to Italy one last time. Which, as they say, is another story.

Also includes chapters on the idiosyncrasies of the Italian language and the Italian driving experience.

Scratching the toe of Italy
Expecting the unexpected in Calabria

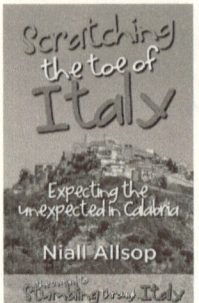

In July 2008 Niall Allsop and his wife Kay returned to the UK after their third holiday in Calabria near the small hill-top town of Santa Severina; the plan was to return the following summer.

Ten weeks later, their left-hand drive Renault Clio bursting at the seams, they left their home in south-west England and headed for the coast on the first leg of their journey back to Calabria to live.

Scratching the toe of Italy continues the story from where *Stumbling through Italy* left off and explains how their move to Italy came about, the logistics of the move itself and what happened next.

It is the story of two adventurous pensioners adapting to being the only English-speaking people in a small Calabrian town, of the new friends they made and the home they created there.

Scratching the toe of Italy is a heart-warming chronicle of perseverance and optimism, of the struggle to come to grips with a new language and a new culture, of starting each day with the certain knowledge that it will not turn out as expected.

Keeping up with the Lawrences
Sicily, Sea and Sardinia revisited

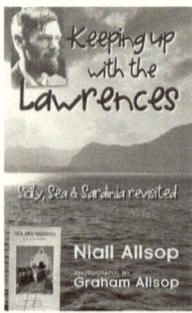

In January 1921 DH Lawrence and his wife, Frieda, left their Taormina home in north-east Sicily and set off on a nine-day excursion to and through Sardinia and back to Sicily via mainland Italy. Lawrence's account of their journey, *Sea and Sardinia*, was published later that year in New York.

Keeping up with the Lawrences is a contemporary account of making the same journey, as far as possible keeping to the same route, the same time scale, the same mode of transport and the same overnight stops as Lawrence and the queen-bee, his pet name for Frieda.

Like *Sea and Sardinia*, *Keeping up with the Lawrences* is written in the present tense but there the comparisons end for the irascible Lawrence was not a tolerant traveller, was not what the Italians would call *simpatico*.

Lawrence travelled at a time of heightened tensions in Europe after the Great War and these are reflected in his outlook and the people he encountered, most of whom he gave appropriate nicknames such as Hamlet, the Bounder, Mr Rochester and the Sludge Queen.

Niall Allsop and his nephew traversed the same route in a different world, a brave new world of iPods and tele-communications masts, and here they met Julius Caesar and Cicero, Wonderwoman, Red and Mr Irritable ... and many more colorful and interesting characters brought to life on the pages of this unique travelogue.

A taste of Calabria

140 Recipes from Southern Italy by Salvatore Vona
Translated by Niall Allsop

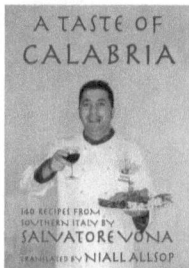

Salvatore Vona is the chef at Le Puzelle, an *agriturismo* (converted farmhouse accommodation) near the small hill-top town of Santa Severina in the Calabrian province of Crotone.

As well as providing holiday accommodation, Le Puzelle is well-known locally for its cuisine and many Calabrians and others travel considerable distances to wine and dine at Salvatore Vona's table.

Salvatore's book of recipes, *A Taste of Calabria*, began life as the third edition of his popular *I Sapori delle Puzelle* (literally the tastes and flavours of the Puzelle) and reflects the demand, expressed by many of Le Puzelle's English-speaking guests, for an English language edition.

Heads will roll

The true story of corruption, conspiracy and confrontation in an English Primary School

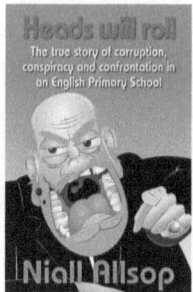

In January 1971 a young, inexperienced teacher took up his position as Deputy Head of a Primary School in a small commuter-belt village not far from London. The School was not what Nigel Allsop (as he was known at the time) was expecting.

The Head of St Patrick's, George Snaith, was involved in a number of unorthodox and illegal practices, only one of which is the focus of this book.

In March that year Allsop witnessed Snaith helping two children during a crucial exam and realized also that the same children had clearly had unauthorized access to the detail of the papers.

Heads will roll is the story of how Nigel Allsop and his teaching colleagues went head to head with Snaith and those in authority who had turned a blind eye to such practices at the school for years.